Tardive Dyskinesia and Affective Disorders

CLINICAL INSIGHTS

Tardive Dyskinesia and Affective Disorders

Edited by
GEORGE GARDOS, MD

Psychiatrist, West-Ros-Park Mental Health Center; and Lecturer on Psychiatry, Harvard Medical School

DANIEL E. CASEY, MD

Clinical Investigator, Medical Research, Psychiatry, and Neurology Services, V.A. Medical Center, Portland; Associate Professor, Departments of Psychiatry and Neurology, Oregon Health Sciences University; and Affiliate Scientist, Oregon Regional Primate Research Center

AMERICAN PSYCHIATRIC PRESS, INC.
Washington, D.C.

Note: The authors have worked to ensure that all information in this book concerning drug dosages, schedules, and routes of administration is accurate at the time of publication and consistent with standards set by the U.S. Food and Drug Administration and the general medical community. As medical research and practice advance, however, therapeutic standards may change. For this reason and because human and mechanical errors sometimes occur, we recommend that readers follow the advice of a physician directly involved in their care or the care of a member of their family.

This monograph is based on material presented at the 136th Annual Meeting of the American Psychiatric Association. That meeting and this monograph are endeavors to share scientific findings and new ideas. The opinions expressed in this monograph are those of the individual authors and not necessarily those of the American Psychiatric Association.

Library of Congress Cataloging in Publication Data

Main entry under title:

Tardive dyskinesia and affective disorders.

(Clinical insights)
Papers presented as a symposium at the 136th Annual Meeting of the American Psychiatric Association, held Apr. 30-May 6, 1983 in New York City.
Includes bibliographies.
1. Tardive dyskinesia—Congresses. 2. Affective disorders—Chemotherapy—Congresses. I. Gardos, George. II. Casey, Daniel E. III. American Psychiatric Association. Meeting
(136th : 1983 : New York, N.Y.) IV. Series. [DNLM: 1. Dyskinesia, Drug-induced—Complications—Congresses. 2. Affective disorders, Psychotic—Complications—Congresses. 3. Tranquilizing agents—Therapeutic use—Congresses. WL 390 T1815 1983]
RC394.T37T35 1984 616.8′3 84-6166
ISBN 0-88048-060-2 (pbk.)

Printed in the U.S.A.

Contents

Contributors

Murray Alpert, PhD
Professor and Director of Psychology, Department of Psychiatry, New York University Medical Center

Michael Bird, AB
Psychopharmacology Program, McLean Hospital

Michael Borenstein, PhD
Department of Psychiatry, Long Island Jewish–Hillside Medical Center

Daniel E. Casey, MD
Clinical Investigator, Medical Research, Psychiatry, and Neurology Services, VA Medical Center, Portland, Oregon; Associate Professor, Departments of Psychiatry and Neurology, Oregon Health Sciences University; and Affiliate Scientist, Oregon Regional Primate Research Center

Jonathan O. Cole, MD
Chief, Psychopharmacology Program, McLean Hospital

George Gardos, MD
Psychiatrist, West-Ros-Park Mental Health Center; and Lecturer on Psychiatry, Harvard Medical School

Joel Gelernter, MD
State University of New York at Stony Brook

David Haskell, MD
Psychiatrist, Veterans Administration Clinic, Boston

John M. Kane, MD
Department of Psychiatry, Long Island Jewish–Hillside Medical Center

Bruce Kinon, MD
Department of Psychiatry, Long Island Jewish–Hillside Medical Center

Jeffrey Lieberman, MD
Department of Psychiatry, Long Island Jewish–Hillside Medical Center

Patricia Moore, RN, MPH
Boston Mental Health Foundation

ROBERT M. RAPKIN, MD
Private Practice, Guilford, Connecticut

ALAN ROSENBAUM, MD
Private Practice, Southfield, Michigan

MICHAEL RUSH, PHD
Clinical Instructor, Department of Psychiatry, New York University Medical Center

SUSAN SCHNIEBOLK, BA
Psychopharmacology Program, McLean Hospital

PAUL WEINHOLD, PHD
Department of Psychiatry, Long Island Jewish–Hillside Medical Center

MARGARET WOERNER, PHD
Department of Psychiatry, Long Island Jewish–Hillside Medical Center

Introduction

At first sight it may appear strange to see two such apparently unrelated conditions joined together in one title. That real links may exist both from the clinical and the neuropharmacological perspectives emerges from the five papers that make up this monograph and which were presented as a symposium at the 136th Annual Meeting of the American Psychiatric Association. The rationale for this topic arose from clinical observations suggesting that neuroleptic-treated patients who suffer either from affective disorders or have significant affective component in their psychotic illness may be at increased risk for developing tardive dyskinesia (TD). If affective disorder indeed emerges as a risk factor in TD, then the employment of neuroleptics in all patients carrying a definite or probable diagnosis falling into the affective disorder spectrum will require careful scrutiny. Understanding the neuropharmacological mechanisms underlying the possible association between TD and affective illness is also undoubtedly of interest to researchers attempting to elucidate the biochemistry and neuropharmacology of depression and mania.

This monograph discusses the accumulating research data relevant to the association between TD and affective illness, and presents studies concerning epidemiology and treatment. Dr. Daniel E. Casey reviews the literature reporting associations between affective disorders and TD. Possible mechanisms of actions are discussed, and specific patient variables (age, sex, other neurological symptoms, TD severity, and mania versus depression) and treatment parameters (neuroleptic dose, duration of treatment, and concomitant drug prescription) are examined. Guidelines for using neuroleptics to treat affective disorders are also reviewed.

Dr. John M. Kane and his colleagues present data from their prospective study of TD development. They found higher incidence and severity of TD in patients with affective disorders as compared to those with schizophrenia. Particularly noteworthy from the clinical standpoint is their finding that the majority of patients who developed TD with less than one year of neuroleptic exposure carried a Research Diagnostic Criteria (RDC) diagnosis of major affective disorder.

Drs. Murray Alpert and Michael Rush present a retrospective study comparing matched groups of patients with and without TD. They found that an increased rate of depression preceded the development of TD. In an attempt to explain their findings, they speculate that depressed patients may be more prone to developing catecholamine receptor hypersensitivity and hence show greater risk for developing TD.

Dr. Alan Rosenbaum presents neuroendocrine data on a small group of depressed patients also suffering from TD. Such patients show unusual clinical features and tend not to respond clinically to antidepressants alone. However, a combination of lithium and tricyclic antidepressants appears to confer benefit on both depression and dyskinesia. The improvement in dyskinesia may appear more slowly (two to four months) than the antidepressant effect.

Dr. Jonathan O. Cole and associates focus on the role of lithium in TD. A review of the literature suggests an important although secondary role in its treatment of schizophrenia when compared to the neuroleptic drugs. The possible role of lithium in the treatment of TD remains uncertain. A study of moderately severe TD is presented in which lithium was significantly superior to placebo during the first eight weeks. However, the lithium-placebo differences were not maintained in the extended study when neuroleptic dosage was tapered.

What are the implications of this monograph for the practicing psychiatrist? Even at this preliminary stage of the research into the association between TD and affective disorders, a few conclusions may be clearly stated. The administration of neuroleptics to patients with affective disorders should not be undertaken lightly. In view of the likelihood of increased risk of TD in such patients, the risk-benefit ratio needs to be carefully considered. Unfortunately, the real world of difficult clinical situations with suicidal, dangerous, excited, and grossly psychotic patients who do not respond to antidepressants or lithium may necessitate the administration of neuroleptics, at least for a limited time, for lack of a suitable alternative. Hence, the problem of TD in the neuroleptic-treated affective patient is likely to stay with us. However, we believe that forewarned may indeed be forearmed, and awareness of the problem may lead to stricter criteria of neuroleptic use and, hopefully, to reduced incidence of TD.

The other finding to emerge from this monograph concerns the role of lithium. Although this drug may have a role in the treatment of TD, either in affective disorders or in schizophrenia, its promise as a possible replacement for neuroleptics in the maintenance treatment of schizophrenics has not been realized. This latter finding is particularly unfortunate since the best way to obviate the problem of TD in both schizophrenics and affective disorder patients is to avoid neuroleptics. At the present state of knowledge, neither lithium nor any other compound has proved to be a satisfactory substitute for neuroleptics. By raising a red flag in the neuroleptic treatment of affective disorder patients, this monograph may serve a useful purpose. However, we hope that an even greater benefit may ultimately accrue from this work if it stimulates research toward novel approaches to the treatment of affective illness and toward the discovery of effective non-neuroleptic antipsychotics.

George Gardos, M.D.
Daniel E. Casey, M.D.

1

Tardive Dyskinesia and Affective Disorders

Daniel E. Casey, M.D.

1

Tardive Dyskinesia and Affective Disorders

Tardive dyskinesia, a potentially irreversible, drug-induced neurological syndrome of abnormal involuntary movements, has caused substantial concern about the proper role of neuroleptic medication use in current-day psychiatric practices. The broad and generalized use of these otherwise relatively safe and highly effective drugs for controlling psychotic symptoms indicates the potential magnitude of the problem. Emphasis is now being placed on identifying appropriate indications for neuroleptic compounds to achieve the maximum benefit with a minimum risk. For patients who benefit only from neuroleptics, these drugs are essential. For patients who are successfully managed with other treatment approaches, neuroleptic use is questionable. The goal, then, is to identify factors which will enable clinicians to assess more accurately the potential benefits and problems of treatment.

In addition to advancing age and perhaps higher risk for females, affective disorders may be another risk factor for tardive dyskinesia. Multiple reports, which will be summarized below, consistently suggest that this may be the case. One study specifically designed to identify a group of patients at high risk for tardive dyskinesia evaluated all of their patients who developed this disorder with less than one year of neuroleptic treatment (Kane et al. 1980). Of the seven patients who met their criteria, five had clear-cut affective disorders. Because affective disorders—particularly depression—are more frequently diagnosed in women in mid- or later life, these three factors may have cumulative effects to further increase the vulnerability to tardive dyskinesia.

The possibility of neuroleptic-induced side effects emphasizes the importance of a thorough clinical evaluation and diagnostic precision. For the few affective disorder patients who are poorly responsive to lithium or antidepressants, neuroleptics should be used for the shortest period of time at the lowest effective dose. New approaches to unmanageable manic-depressive illness, such as treatment with carbamazepine (Tegretol), should also be given careful consideration (Post 1982).

The aim of this chapter is to review our current knowledge about the relationship between tardive dyskinesia and affective disorders. Findings about mood-dependent dyskinesias, the role of lithium in preventing tardive dyskinesia, and the possible effect of tardive dyskinesia on cognitive and mood lability will be examined. Therapeutic strategies which suggest that effectively treating the underlying affective disorder may also substantially ameliorate tardive dyskinesia will also be summarized. Finally, the guidelines for neuroleptic use from the American Psychiatric Association Task Force Report on Tardive Dyskinesia (1980) will be reviewed with particular reference to affective disorders.

IS AFFECTIVE DISORDER A RISK FACTOR FOR TARDIVE DYSKINESIA?

The question of whether affective disorders increase the risk of developing tardive dyskinesia is receiving increasing attention. The final answer will have to await the outcome of extended prospective studies with groups well matched for patient characteristics, diagnosis, and treatment. In the interim, the issue can be addressed by reviewing data from the few available reports. While firm conclusions cannot yet be drawn, some of the general patterns that emerge can guide clinical practice and direct future research.

The reported prevalence rates of tardive dyskinesia in patients

Table 1 Tardive Dyskinesia in Affective Disorders: Selected Samples

Author	Year	Patients*	Prevalence	Comments
Davis et al.	1976	9/14	64%	Depression common; previous diagnosis of schizophrenia
Rosenbaum et al.	1977	9/12	75%	Depression common in retrospective chart review
		15/18	83%	Depression common in 18 consecutive TD cases in prospective study
Kane et al.	1980	5/7	71%	From 99 consecutive TD cases, high-risk group: TD in <1 year neuroleptic treatment
Rush et al.	1982	7/11	64%	Mood disorder symptoms high at first hospitalization when diagnosed schizophrenia; 7 rediagnosed as affective disorder
Hamra et al.	1983	12/17	71%	Included both affective disorders and paranoid schizophrenia; more TD in older females
Yassa et al.	1983	34/83	41%	Affective disorders program included "atypical" schizophrenia; more TD in older patients
Casey and Toenniessen	1984	8/27	30%	Outpatient TD clinic; 8 schizophrenic patients rediagnosed as affective disorder

*Data are the numbers of patients with affective disorders and tardive dyskinesia/total studied. TD = tardive dyskinesia.

with affective disorders are summarized in Table 1. These rates, which range from 30 to 83 percent, exceed the broad range of 0 to 56 percent reported for tardive dyskinesia in the past 20 years (Kane and Smith 1982). To further clarify whether these higher rates reflect increased vulnerability or are artifactually high in these selected samples, prevalence rates will have to be compared with other matched controlled populations at risk for tardive dyskinesia, such as schizophrenia (see Chapter 2 of this monograph).

Three of the reports in Table 1 identify a high rate of depression in patients with tardive dyskinesia (Davis et al. 1976; Rosenbaum et al. 1977; Rush et al. 1982). Although the other studies do not specifically examine this issue, the clinical data may not have been available. These reports also focus attention on the accuracy of psychiatric diagnosis. In two studies, the majority of patients with a current diagnosis of affective disorder and tardive dyskinesia were previously diagnosed as schizophrenic (Davis et al. 1976; Rush et al. 1982). When this issue was specifically studied, patients with descriptions of abnormal mood and a diagnosis of schizophrenia at the time of their first hospitalization were more likely to develop tardive dyskinesia, and upon further evaluation failed to meet the criteria for a diagnosis of schizophrenia (Rush et al. 1982). (For a more in-depth discussion of this issue, see Chapter 3 of this monograph.) In the two patient samples evaluated by Rosenbaum et al. (1977), the large majority of patients also suffered from depression. Though a few of these patients with "tardive dyskinesia" may not have had this disorder because they had not received prior neuroleptic treatment (as required by the definition of tardive dyskinesia), the observation of hyperkinetic abnormal movements in patients with depression is striking.

In studies that do not control for psychiatric diagnosis, advancing age is consistently associated with increased prevalence of tardive dyskinesia. One study large enough to look at this question in patients with affective disorders did find that those with tardive dyskinesia were older than those without this syndrome. Unfortunately, too little information is available to compare accurately specific tardive dyskinesia prevalence rates by psychiatric diagnosis, so it is not yet possible to know whether potential risk factors such as age and affective disorders are cumulative.

Most studies evaluating the relationship between gender and tardive dyskinesia conclude that females are at high risk (Kane and Smith 1982). The question of whether or not affective disorders additionally increase the risk for tardive dyskinesia deserves careful evaluation. This concern is especially warranted because women are more likely to be diagnosed as "depressed" and "mood disordered" and to be treated with psychopharmacological agents—including neuroleptics.

The consensus of findings shows no relationship between the drug treatment parameters of dose, duration, or type of neuroleptic and tardive dyskinesia. There are a few notable exceptions, however, that do report a significant relationship between duration of treatment and tardive dyskinesia in the elderly when treatment is limited to less than a few years (Toenniessen et al. 1984). This study identified a strong association between tardive dyskinesia and duration of treatment for the first three years of drug therapy, but no such relationship existed for the subsequent 20 years of treatment. This suggests, at least in the elderly, a period of maximum vulnerability for developing tardive dyskinesia. If this concept can be applied to other risk factors, patients with affective disorders may also have a period of maximum vulnerability to tardive dyskinesia. When in the course of treatment this risk is greatest is as yet unknown, but it may also occur in the early phases of neuroleptic exposure (less than three years). This possibility is hinted at in case reports that observe some of the most severe cases of tardive dyskinesia occur in patients with affective disorders and relatively brief durations of neuroleptic treatment. Though these observations are anecdotal, the possibility of such an association further argues for the cautious use of neuroleptic drugs in affective disorder patients.

Possible Mechanisms

If the risk of tardive dyskinesia is greater in affective disorders, it will be necessary to explain how this increased risk might occur. The most parsimonious explanations will have to involve at least partially overlapping mechanisms that underlie the pathogenesis and/or pathophysiology of these disorders. Because these disorders are incompletely understood, any hypothesis offered will undoubtedly be oversimplified (Table 2).

The mechanism of interacting processes related to disease states and treatment effects offered by Davis et al. (1976) to explain their findings of increased depression in patients with tardive dyskinesia

Table 2 Affective Disorders and Risk of Tardive Dyskinesia: Possible Interacting Mechanisms

Mood/Treatment	CNS Amine Activity	Change in CNS Sensitivity
Depression	Decreased	Supersensitivity NE, SER; ?DA
Mania	Increased	Subsensitivity NE, SER; ?DA
Neuroleptics	Decreased	Supersensitivity DA; ?NE, ?SER
Antidepressants	Increased	Subsensitivity NE, SER; ?DA
Lithium	Stabilized	Stabilize

Abbreviations: CNS = central nervous system, NE = norepinephrine, SER = serotonin, DA = dopamine.

is intrinsically appealing. Decreased aminergic activity, whether it be the indolamine serotonin or the catecholamines norepinephrine and dopamine, has been proposed as the fundamental neurotransmitter alteration underlying depression. This decreased neurotransmitter activity could result in a "chemical denervation" and lead to increased postsynaptic sensitivity. Neuroleptic drugs, which preferentially block dopamine receptors, but also influence other amines, could similarly lead to a state of chemical denervation. Treating depressed patients with neuroleptic drugs could then lead to a combination of decreased neurotransmitter activity and receptor blockade that would more likely produce receptor supersensitivity.

Extending this line of reasoning to the manic state, the hypothesized increased influence of norepinephrine, serotonin, or possibly dopamine could lead to subsensitivity. Treatment with neuroleptic drugs at this time would possibly be less likely to produce supersensitivity because there would be compensating mechanisms of sub- and supersensitivity. Carrying this model further, antidepressant treatment, which purportedly induces catecholamine subsensitivity, might be able to compensate, at least in part, for neuroleptic-induced supersensitivity. Finally, lithium, whose mechanism of action is incompletely understood but perhaps works via mechanisms of membrane stabilization, might be able to foster or maintain homeostatic processes to reduce both mood swings and possibly the risk of treatment-induced central nervous system (CNS) changes.

In animal models, lithium has been shown to prevent the development of dopamine receptor hypersensitivity in both behavorial and biochemical parameters (Klawans et al. 1977; Pert et al. 1978). It is theoretically intriguing to ask whether a combination of lithium plus neuroleptic treatment in the clinic would also prevent the development of tardive dyskinesia. To date, there are no data to answer this question, but it may be a potentially worthwhile line of investigation.

Other questions naturally arise from these undoubtedly oversimplified mechanistic explanations of interacting influences of disease and treatment. This schematic approach implies that using neuroleptic drugs during a depressive phase would be more likely to produce tardive dyskinesia than would using neuroleptics in acute mania. It could also be argued that patients with unipolar depressive syndromes may be most at risk for tardive dyskinesia if they receive neuroleptic drugs, whereas bipolar patients or unipolar manics may have less risk. Until data bear out or refute these considerations, using neuroleptic drugs for extended periods of time in psychotic delusional depressions or to control mania will need to be carefully balanced with the potential risks.

A separate mechanism of cycling mood states as a model of kindling may suggest an increased risk of tardive dyskinesia in affective disorders. The repeated cycling of moods could lead to—or perhaps is reflective of—increased CNS lability and therefore increase the vulnerability either to disease or treatment-induced receptor or neurotransmitter effects.

MOOD-DEPENDENT DYSKINESIAS

Mood-dependent, also called state-dependent, dyskinesias have been observed rarely in a few patients who experience dramatic changes in symptoms of tardive dyskinesia during mood changes (Cutler et al. 1981; Applebaum 1982; Weiner and Werner 1982;

DePotter et al. 1983; Linnoila et al. 1983). All of these patients, except for one with unipolar depression, suffered from rapid-cycling, bipolar manic-depressive illness, and shared the characteristic of decreased tardive dyskinesia during mania. Most of these patients also had an aggravation of tardive dyskinesia during depression. In the euthymic state, tardive dyskinesia may or may not have been present in these different patients. A few case reports documented that the changes in tardive dyskinesia preceded the changes in mood state by a few days to a few weeks (Cutler and Post 1982; Weiner and Werner 1982). These reports also noted that most of the patients were poorly responsive to the usual pharmacological approaches to manic-depressive illness. At least two of these patients developed tardive dyskinesia with relatively short durations of neuroleptic treatment of less than three years (Weiner and Werner 1982; DePotter et al. 1983). Because only a few patients have been reported, it is not possible to assess if there is a gender vulnerability to this syndrome. The majority of reports do not have sufficient data to clarify the eventual outcome of this disorder, but one patient had his tardive dyskinesia resolve at least two years after its onset during a trial of carbamazepine (Tegretol) (Cutler and Post 1982). Whether this is related to the drug treatment or to the natural history of slowly reversible tardive dyskinesia is unclear (Casey and Toenniessen 1984).

Biochemical data about the mechanisms underlying these mood-dependent dyskinesias are sketchy. In one patient, norepinephrine and gamma aminobutyric acid (GABA) concentrations in the cerebrospinal fluid were significantly increased in mania, compared to depression, whereas the dopamine metabolite homovanillic acid and the serotonin metabolite 5-hydroxyindole acetic acid did not significantly differ according to mood phase (Cutler and Post 1982). In another biochemical evaluation, urinary phenylethylamine, a purported endogenous amphetamine-like amine, was significantly increased in both mania and depression, but the magnitude was greater in the depressive phase (Linnoila et al. 1983). The authors speculated that phenylethylamine was not causally related to the changes in tardive dyskinesia because two patients had equally high urinary phenylethylamine levels during both manic and depressive cycles.

These mood-dependent dyskinesias appeared to change in ways that conflict with what might be expected from the mechanisms proposed in the previous section. According to the "classic" hypotheses, mania is associated with a relative increase in amine activity that should further activate the supersensitive dopamine receptors underlying tardive dyskinesia. Conversely, depression should lead to a decrease in dyskinetic symptoms. The findings with these mood-dependent dyskinesias obviously do not conform to this framework. Rather, the clinical observations are opposite to what would be predicted. However, some caveats should be offered. The majority of patients with affective disorders and tardive dyskinesia do not seem to be characterized by a mood-dependent status of their dyskinesias, though it is unclear what percentage of these patients do experience state-dependent changes. Patients with this mood-dependent disorder may be the exceptions, not the rule. On the other hand, this phenomenon may occur quite commonly but has only been noted as a casual clinical observation, such as the brief mention of two patients whose dyskinesia became worse during depression (Rosenbaum et al. 1977). In either case, these clinical observations seem to identify a subgroup of patients (e.g., rapid cyclers, poor responders to treatment, mood-dependent dyskinesias), which may provide important data about the pathophysiological mechanisms underlying these disorders.

Though there are obviously too few data to offer satisfactory explanations of how these disorders may interact, the findings of mood-dependent dyskinesias raise important questions about the underlying pathophysiological mechanisms. Affective disorders may not be explained primarily by perturbations of norepinephrine and serotonin. Similarly, tardive dyskinesia may not be explained primarily on the basis of supersensitive dopamine receptors. A variety of mechanisms including, but not limited to, purported imbalances between multiple subtypes of receptors, sub-

and supersensitivity, and other neurotransmitters could be offered as speculative explanations of this disorder.

TREATMENT

Observations made during attempts to treat these coexisting syndromes further confirm important relationships between affective disorders and tardive dyskinesia. In one study of 19 patients with depression and tardive dyskinesia, 11 (58 percent) showed marked or moderate decreases in tardive dyskinesia and improvement in mood with tricyclic antidepressants and lithium over one to two months of treatment (Rosenbaum et al. 1980a). Four patients not receiving antidepressant therapy were also followed and showed no change in tardive dyskinesia. While it is possible that some of the patients who improved were experiencing the natural resolution of slowly reversible tardive dyskinesia, this cannot be a suitable explanation for all patients because a few discontinued medications and had relapses of both their depression and tardive dyskinesia. It was also the investigators' opinion that tricyclic antidepressants and lithium were more effective in combined therapy than if either of the compounds was used alone. One of the few patients with mood-dependent dyskinesias who failed to respond to the usual forms of drug treatment for depression did benefit from a trial of carbamazepine by showing an improvement in mood and a resolution of tardive dyskinesia (Cutler and Post 1982). This patient also may have experienced a spontaneous resolution of tardive dyskinesia, but the fairly prompt improvement of symptoms after two years of relatively stable tardive dyskinesia suggests the drug treatment may have had at least some influence.

Information about the effect of electroconvulsive therapy (ECT) in affective disorders comes from case reports (Asnis and Leopold 1978; Price and Levin 1978; Rosenbaum et al. 1980b). One patient improved with ECT (Price and Levin 1978) and another showed similar benefit from ECT and continuing tricyclic antidepressant plus lithium therapy during the six-month follow-up (Rosenbaum et al. 1980b). Conflicting observations come from a report of four patients whose mental status improved with ECT, but showed no consistent change in tardive dyskinesia (Asnis and Leopold 1978).

The effect of lithium as a treatment for tardive dyskinesia has been the subject of conflicting reports (for review and new data, see chapter by Cole et al.). Though the initial reports about lithium and tardive dyskinesia were enthusiastic, the later studies found no consistent benefit and even occasional aggravation of symptoms. Perhaps the positive results in previous studies are related to the inclusion of a few patients with depression that was responsive to lithium, whereas the majority of patients in these studies were euthymic or suffered from other psychiatric illnesses such as schizophrenia.

OTHER NEUROLOGICAL RELATIONSHIPS

Recently, a few studies have addressed the relationship between affective disorder and tardive dyskinesia by evaluating whether other neurological changes are observable in patients with these two syndromes. The focus of these inquiries is to ask whether those variables which cause tardive dyskinesia, or tardive dyskinesia itself, can cause other specific neurological dysfunction. The issue of cognitive function and tardive dyskinesia is an area of obvious relevance. Whether organic brain syndromes are a risk factor for developing tardive dyskinesia is unclear. Data for and against this hypothesis have been presented and summarized (Kane and Smith 1982). In a review of studies evaluating the spontaneous dyskinesias that resemble tardive dyskinesia, organic brain disease was a significant risk factor for developing spontaneous dyskinesias, particularly in the older patients (Casey and Hansen 1984).

One study examining the relationships between affective disorder, tardive dyskinesia, and cognitive function compared multiple aspects of intellectual performance in patients with schizophrenia and affective disorders with and without tardive dyskinesia (Wolf et al. 1983). A series of neuropsychological assessments were given to each group (eight schizophrenic patients with or without tardive dyskinesia; six affective disorder patients with and without tardive dyskinesia). The patients with tardive dyskinesia and affective disorders had significantly lower scores than affective disorder patients without tardive dyskinesia. There were no differences between the schizophrenic groups with or without tardive dyskinesia. The authors point out that these interesting observations may have existed prior to treatment and the onset of tardive dyskinesia, so the results must be interpreted cautiously. In future efforts to replicate these findings, it will also be important to control for both equally matched past and current drug treatments and mood status in each group, because it has been suggested that lithium and neuroleptics, as well as depression, may temporarily impair cognitive abilities.

A separate line of study suggests that tardive dyskinesia may be associated with a newly defined syndrome, "tardive dysmentia," characterized by changes in affect, activation level, and interpersonal interaction (Wilson et al. 1983). It is hypothesized that those factors which cause tardive dyskinesia may also be causing other neurological changes in the CNS, particularly alterations in affect. This proposal was investigated in 29 schizophrenic patients, all of whom had tardive dyskinesia. The mean length of hospitalization was 16.8 years, and the mean length of neuroleptic treatment was 17 years. The authors were confident that the diagnosis of schizophrenia was accurate and that their findings could not be explained on the basis of misdiagnosed affective disorders. The results from an interview and rating of abnormal movements with the Abnormal Involuntary Movement Scale (AIMS) showed a significant positive correlation between severity of tardive dyskinesia and symptoms of unstable mood, loud speech, and approach to the examiner.

These interesting observations should stimulate further study and attempts at replication. The provocative implication of this hypothesis and preliminary finding is that there may be a phenomenon of "tardive affective disorder," which might be akin to the proposed but yet-to-be verified "tardive psychosis" or "supersensitivity psychosis" (Davis and Rosenberg 1979; Chouinard and Jones 1980). Other explanations, however, must be considered, and additional studies need to control for many potentially confounding variables before tardive dysmentia is substantiated. Drug treatment, both past and current, must be balanced in matched samples for further study. Current neuroleptic dose may be particularly relevant, as higher doses can mask existing tardive dyskinesia and successfully control psychotic symptoms. Conversely, patients on low doses or no neuroleptic drugs may have their tardive dyskinesia and psychosis unmasked.

The effects of institutionalization must also be closely examined. These patients, who had been hospitalized for an average of almost 17 years, undoubtedly developed some deviant behaviors due to long-term institutionalization. Furthermore, these patients may not be representative of the typical population receiving neuroleptics. Because these patients were unable to be discharged from the hospital, they may have had a subtype of psychosis that was poorly responsive to treatment and therefore suffered from other underlying neurological dysfunction. Finally, these observations must be considered within the context of the natural history of chronic psychosis. In the era prior to pharmacological treatment, subgroups of both schizophrenia and affective disorders had a course of progressive deterioration characterized by severe chronic psychosis that may have been accompanied by spontaneously occurring involuntary movements resembling drug-induced tardive dyskinesia (Kraepelin 1907; Casey and Hansen 1984).

Guidelines for Neuroleptic Use in Affective Disorders

The possibility that affective disorders may be a risk factor for tardive dyskinesia argues for cautious and careful use of neuroleptic drugs in patients with mood disorders. Though these drugs are commonly used to manage affective symptoms, such treatment practices are based more on clinical experience than on a broad base of scientific knowledge. Schizophrenia is the only disorder for which the long-term use of neuroleptic drugs has been convincingly demonstrated. In the absence of data about the role of neuroleptics for treating affective disorders, heeding the guidelines

Table 3 Indications for Use of Neuroleptics in Affective Disorders

Short-Term Use
- Acute psychotic episodes
- Acute reduction of manic-excitement when the onset of lithium's effect is too slow
- Adjunctive therapy for psychotic depressions when antidepressants or ECT may not be successful

Long-Term Use
Secondary Indications
- Extremely unstable manic-depressive symptoms or other episodic psychoses (rare)

Questionable Indications
- Recurrent mood disorders

NOTE. Adapted from the Task Force Report on Tardive Dyskinesia (American Psychiatric Association 1980).

of the American Psychiatric Association Task Force Report on Tardive Dyskinesia (1980) (Table 3) should stand the clinician in good stead.

Indications for using neuroleptics in the short term, defined as approximately six months or less, are tailored to manage acute psychosis effectively. Since tardive dyskinesia has very rarely been shown to occur within this relatively brief time frame, the risk should be minimized by limiting treatment to this duration. According to the Task Force Report on Tardive Dyskinesia, the primary indications for short-term use of neuroleptic drugs are (1) acute psychotic episodes; (2) acute reduction of manic excitement when the onset of lithium's effect is too slow; and (3) adjunctive therapy for psychotic depression when antidepressants or ECT alone may not be successful.

The long-term use of neuroleptic drugs in affective disorders is debatable. None of the recommended primary indications for the appropriate extended use of these drugs in the Task Force Report is related to affective disorders. One of the justified secondary indications is extremely unstable manic-depressive psychosis. This phenomenon, however, is relatively rare and does not apply to typical manic-depressive disorders. The Task Force recognizes under the category of questionable indications that these drugs are used in recurrent mood disorders, but neither the efficacy nor the safety of this approach has been adequately demonstrated in controlled studies. The intent of the Task Force Report is to emphasize that most patients with affective disorders will not need to take neuroleptic drugs for prolonged periods. In those uncommon patients who do need to take these drugs to maintain clinical stability, a conservative approach is warranted. This can best be achieved by using the lowest effective dose for the shortest length of time only in those patients who have chronic symptoms that are responsive to treatment.

CONCLUSIONS

Evidence from multiple lines of study suggests that affective disorders may be a risk factor for developing tardive dyskinesia. The few epidemiological studies of selected patient samples with tardive dyskinesia found high rates of affective disorders, particularly depression. Since many of these patients were retrospectively rediagnosed as affective disorders from previous diagnoses of schizophrenia, the importance of initial diagnostic accuracy is emphasized. Mechanisms that might account for this proposed increased vulnerability have been suggested. Perhaps alterations in CNS amine activity during mood changes, coupled with changes induced by drug treatment, produce cumulative or counteracting effects. Mood-dependent dyskinesias, though rare, have been reported in a few rapid-cycling patients who were poorly responsive to standard forms of treatment. These observations of increased tardive dyskinesia with depression and resolution of symptoms in mania may give insights into the pathophysiology underlying both the mood and movement disorders. Antidepressant and lithium therapy may be effective in treating both tardive dyskinesia and depression in some patients. The possibility that these disorders are also associated with other neurological dysfunction, such as cognitive impairment or tardive dyskinesia, requires further study.

The suggestive evidence of affective disorders as a risk factor for tardive dyskinesia adds further caution to the appropriately conservative indications for using neuroleptics. In the short term, the use of these drugs should be limited to managing acute psychotic symptoms. In the long term, the use of neuroleptic drugs in affective disorders should be reserved for manic-depressive illness that is not responsive to standard therapy. The goal is to use the lowest effective dose for the shortest period of time in patients who are known responders to neuroleptics. Alternative drug treatments such as carbamazepine for the unstable manic-depressive patient are under active investigation and should be considered.

Future research must clarify if affective disorders are indeed a risk factor for tardive dyskinesia. Prospective studies, as well as concurrent investigations with properly matched samples and rigorous designs, will be necessary to identify patients at risk and those who might benefit from different treatment approaches. Until that time, neuroleptic medications for affective disorders should be carefully considered and cautiously prescribed.

References

American Psychiatric Association: Tardive Dyskinesia, Task Force Report No. 18. Washington, DC, American Psychiatric Association, 1980

Applebaum PS: Dyskinesia and unipolar depression. Am J Psychiatry 139:140–141, 1982

Asnis GM, Leopold MA: A single-blind study of ECT in patients with tardive dyskinesia. Am J Psychiatry 135:1235–1237, 1978

Baldessarini RJ, Cole JO, Davis JM, et al: Tardive Dyskinesia: A Task Force Report. Washington, DC, American Psychiatric Association, 1980

Casey DE, Hansen TE: Spontaneous dyskinesia, in Neuropsychiatric Movement Disorders. Edited by Jeste DJ, Wyatt RJ. Washington, DC, American Psychiatric Press, Inc. (in press)

Casey DE, Toenniessen LM: Neuroleptic treatment in tardive dyskinesia: can it be developed into a clinical strategy for long-term treatment? in New Directions in Tardive Dyskinesia Research. Edited by Bannet J, Belmaker RH. Basel, Switzerland, Karger (in press)

Chouinard G, Jones BD: Neuroleptic-induced supersensitivity psychosis: clinical and pharmacologic characteristics. Am J Psychiatry 137:16–21, 1980

Cutler NR, Post RM: State-related cyclical dyskinesias in manic-depressive illness. J Clin Psychopharmacol 2:350–354, 1982

Cutler NR, Post RM, Rey A, et al: Depression-dependent dyskinesias in two cases of manic-depressive illness. N Engl J Med 304:1088–1089, 1981

Davis KL, Rosenberg GS: Is there a limbic system equivalent of tardive dyskinesia? Biol Psychiatry 14:699–703, 1979

Davis KL, Berger PA, Hollister LE: Tardive dyskinesia and depressive illness. Psychopharmacology Communications 2:125–130, 1976

DePotter RW, Linkowski P, Mendlewicz J: State-dependent tardive dyskinesia in manic-depressive illness. J Neurol Neurosurg Psychiatry 46:666–668, 1983

Hamra BJ, Nasrallah HA, Clancy J, et al: Psychiatric diagnosis and risk for tardive dyskinesia. Arch Gen Psychiatry 40:346–347, 1983

Kane JM, Smith JM: Tardive dyskinesia: prevalence and risk factors, 1959 to 1979. Arch Gen Psychiatry 39:473–481, 1982

Kane J, Struve FA, Weinhold P, et al: Strategy for the study of patients at high risk for tardive dyskinesia. Am J Psychiatry 137:1265–1267, 1980

Klawans HL, Weiner WJ, Nausieda PA: The effect of lithium on an animal model of tardive dyskinesia. Prog Neuropsychopharmacol 1:53–60, 1977

Kraepelin E: Clinical Psychiatry. Adapted by Defendorf AR. New York, Macmillan, 1907

Linnoila M, Karoum F, Cutler NR, et al: Temporal association between depression-dependent dyskinesias and high urinary phenylethylamine output. Biol Psychiatry 18:513–516, 1983

Pert A, Rosenblatt JE, Sivit C, et al: Long-term treatment with lithium prevents the development of dopamine receptor supersensitivity. Science 201:171–173, 1978

Post RM: Carbamazepine's acute and prophylactic effects in manic and depressive illness: an update. International Drug Therapy Newsletter 17:5–10, 1982

Price TRP, Levin R: The effects of electroconvulsive therapy on tardive dyskinesia. Am J Psychiatry 135:991, 1978

Rosenbaum AH, Niven RG, Hanson NP, et al: Tardive dyskinesia: relationship with a primary affective disorder. Diseases of the Nervous System 38:423–427, 1977

Rosenbaum AH, Maruta T, Duane DD, et al: Tardive dyskinesia in depressed patients: successful therapy with antidepressants and lithium. Psychosomatics 21:715–719, 1980a

Rosenbaum AH, O'Connor MK, Duane DD, et al: Treatment of tardive dyskinesia in an agitated, depressed patient. Psychosomatics 21:765–766, 1980b

Rush M, Diamond F, Alpert M: Depression as a risk factor in tardive dyskinesia. Biol Psychiatry 17:387–392, 1982

Toenniessen LM, Casey DE, McFarland BH: Tardive dyskinesia in the aged. Arch Gen Psychiatry (in press)

Weiner WJ, Werner TR: Mania-induced remission of tardive dyskinesia in manic-depressive illness. Ann Neurology 12:229–230, 1982

Wilson IC, Garbutt JC, Lanier CF, et al: Is there a tardive dysmentia? Schizophr Bull 9:187–191, 1983

Wolf ME, Ryan JJ, Mosnaim AD: Cognitive functions in tardive dyskinesia. Psychol Med 13:671–674, 1983

Yassa R, Ghadirian AM, Schwartz G: Prevalence of tardive dyskinesia in affective disorder patients. J Clin Psychiatry 44:410–412, 1983

2

Incidence and Severity of Tardive Dyskinesia in Affective Illness

John M. Kane, M.D.
Margaret Woerner, Ph.D.
Paul Weinhold, Ph.D.
Bruce Kinon, M.D.
Jeffrey Lieberman, M.D.
Michael Borenstein, Ph.D.

2

Incidence and Severity of Tardive Dyskinesia in Affective Illness

The identification of risk factors remains an important goal of research in tardive dyskinesia (TD) (Kane and Smith 1980). In the previous chapter, Casey reviewed the existing literature on affective illness as a risk factor. One of the major difficulties in determining the role of diagnosis in predisposing to tardive dyskinesia is the fact that only a portion of patients with affective illness are treated with neuroleptics, and these patients are not necessarily representative of the larger population of patients suffering from these illnesses.

To study this issue, the ideal design would be random assignment to neuroleptics and prospective assessment of patients with schizophrenia and patients with affective illness (matched on other potentially important variables, such as age and sex). Such a study would be problematic on practical and ethical grounds; therefore, we must rely on a variety of naturalistic strategies to address this question.

We have chosen to explore the relationship between a diagnosis of affective illness and three different aspects of tardive dyskinesia: incidence, severity, and persistence.

THREE ASPECTS OF TARDIVE DYSKINESIA

Incidence

To generate information relevant to the incidence of TD in different diagnostic groups, we have drawn on a body of data collected during an ongoing prospective study of tardive dyskinesia development. The methodology of this study has been previously reported (Kane et al. 1982).

Because the patients participating in this study were selected without regard to diagnosis or neuroleptic treatment history, we have had the opportunity to follow a large number of patients with affective illness, some of whom have been treated with neuroleptics.

For the first analysis we used hospital discharge diagnosis [largely DSM-II since this study began before the introduction of DSM-III] and generated life table analyses contrasting the incidence of tardive dyskinesia development per year of neuroleptic exposure for those patients with schizophrenia and those patients with schizoaffective or affective illness (Figure 1). The results

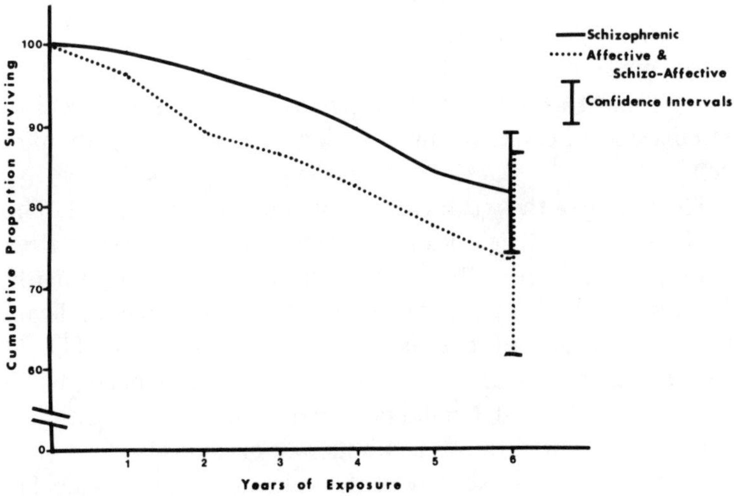

Figure 1 Tardive dyskinesia over six years of neuroleptic exposure by diagnosis.

Table 1 RDC Diagnoses of TD Patients and Matched Controls

Diagnosis	TD (n = 54)	Matched No. TD (n = 54)
Major Affective Disorder	30%	22%
Schizoaffective	24%	9%
Schizophrenia	41%	41%
Other	6%	28%

Statistical Analysis: $\chi^2 = 12.69$; $df = 3$; $p < .01$.

indicate that at the end of six years of cumulative neuroleptic exposure the incidence of tardive dyskinesia is 26% ± 13% for the schizoaffective/affective group compared with 18% ± 7% for the schizophrenia group, a statistically significant difference ($p < .05$ by Lee Desu test). Though these results are suggestive, they must be viewed with caution since other potential risk factors (e.g., age at first treatment, dosage, continuousness of treatment), are not necessarily equal in the two groups.

In addressing some of these concerns, we matched 54 patients who developed presumptive TD during the course of the study with a control group of 54 prospectively followed patients without TD for age, sex, and length of neuroleptic exposure. We compared the matched groups on Research Diagnostic Criteria (RDC) diagnoses, made blind to TD status. Diagnoses were grouped as follows: major affective disorder, schizoaffective disorder, schizophrenia, and other (personality disorders, organic brain syndromes, etc.).

The results of these comparisons are presented in Table 1. The results indicated a significant difference in distribution of diagnoses ($\chi^2 = 12.69$, $p < .01$); however, the difference was primarily the result of a higher proportion of the "other" diagnoses in the no TD group, major affective disorder was similar for the TD (30 percent) and no TD (22 percent) groups. (Fifteen patients with TD could not be matched, but did not differ from the group included in the analysis in terms of distribution of diagnosis.)

Another aspect of risk may be the vulnerability to develop TD with relatively brief cumulative exposure to neuroleptics. We

Table 2 Hospital (DSM-II) Diagnosis and Severity of TD

	Diagnosis			
Most Severe TD Rating	Major Affective Disorder (n = 42)	Schizoaffective (n = 21)	Schizophrenia (n = 96)	Other (n = 28)
Mild	33%	48%	55%	61%
Moderate	38%	43%	39%	25%
Moderately Severe and Very Severe	29%	10%	6%	14%

Statistical Analysis: $\chi^2 = 16.44$; $df = 6$; $p < .02$. ($\chi^2 = 14.04$; $df = 4$; $p < .001$; affective disorder vs schizophrenia).

have previously suggested that patients with affective illness appeared to be overrepresented among those patients developing TD with less than one year of neuroleptic exposure (Kane et al. 1980). Utilizing data from the prospective study, we identified 11 patients who developed TD with less than one year lifetime exposure to neuroleptics and 55 patients who took longer to develop the disorder. Of the "early onset" group, 55 percent had RDC diagnosis of major affective disorder as compared to 22 percent of remaining patients ($\chi^2 = 4.95$, $p < .05$).

Severity

The risk of tardive dyskinesia must be viewed in the context of severity and persistence to achieve the proper perspective. Factors associated with the development of the more severe and/or persistent forms of the disorder have yet to be identified. To explore the relationship between psychiatric diagnosis and severity of TD, we utilized rating scale data on 187 cases of tardive dyskinesia examined by our group over the past six years. We utilized the most severe global TD rating for each patient in comparing severity across diagnostic categories (DSM-II). As can be seen in Table 2, 29 percent of the affective disorder patients had at least one rating of "very severe" as compared to 6 percent of the schizophrenic patients ($\chi^2 = 14.04$, $p < .001$).

Table 3 Severity of TD for Patients Receiving Neuroleptics at Time of Highest TD Rating

	Hospital Diagnosis (DSM-II)	
Highest TD Rating	Major Affective Disorder (n = 14)	Schizophrenia (n = 61)
Mild	36%	62%
Moderate	36%	31%
Moderately Severe/Severe	29%	7%

Statistical Analysis: $\chi^2 = 6.65$; $df = 2$; $p < .05$.

Since the administration of neuroleptics may mask or reduce the severity of the symptoms of TD, we considered the possibility that patients with affective illness were more likely to have been withdrawn from neuroleptics, and, therefore, less likely to have their symptoms partially masked. This might account for the greater proportion of more severe ratings among affective disorders. It turned out that patients with affective illness were significantly more likely than schizophrenics to be off neuroleptics at the time of their highest (most severe) TD rating (58 percent for the affective illness group as compared to 15 percent for the schizophrenia group, $p < .001$). Therefore, we looked at the severity ratings for all TD patients who were receiving neuroleptics at the time of their highest rating and again found a significant relationship between diagnoses and severity, with the affectively ill group receiving the highest ratings (Table 3). When we looked at only those patients who had been withdrawn from neuroleptics, this relationship was not apparent.

The issue of severity after drug withdrawal, however, might be influenced by the length of time patients are followed after drug withdrawal since some improvement might be anticipated following long periods off medication. Therefore, it is necessary to consider persistence in this context as well, and comparisons regarding persistence and severity should involve patients who were systematically assessed at the same intervals following drug withdrawal.

Table 4 RDC Diagnosis and Persistence of TD Among Patients Withdrawn from Medication for at Least Three Months After TD Diagnosis

	RDC–TD Diagnosis	
Diagnosis	Persistent Neuroleptic Free	Transient
Major Affective Disorder (n = 10)	70%	30%
Schizoaffective (n = 3)	67%	33%
Schizophrenia (n = 8)	50%	50%
Other (n = 5)	60%	40%

Persistence

The degree to which tardive dyskinesia persists following withdrawal of neuroleptics varies considerably. In addition, there has not been universal agreement as to what length of time should elapse before the disorder is called "persistent" or "irreversible." The Research Diagnoses for Tardive Dyskinesia suggested by Schooler and Kane (1982) uses a three-month period to define persistence (as long as no reinstitution of neuroleptics or increase in dosage takes place during this interval).

Table 4 presents TD outcome by diagnostic group for those patients who developed TD in the prospective study and who were withdrawn from neuroleptic medication for at least three months following the diagnoses of TD. No significant differences were found on this comparison.

CONCLUSION

In summary, our results thus far provide some support for the role of affective illness as a risk factor in the development of tardive dyskinesia, but the size of the effect appears modest and the data are not consistent. Despite the lack of clear-cut and compelling evidence, it is not premature to suggest considerable caution in the use of neuroleptics for the treatment of patients with affective illness.

References

Kane J, Smith J: Tardive dyskinesia: prevalence and risk factors, 1959–1979. Arch Gen Psychiatry 39:473–481, 1982

Kane J, Struve F, Weinhold P, et al: Strategy for the study of patients at high risk for tardive dyskinesia. Am J Psychiatry 137:1265–1267, 1980

Kane J, Woerner M, Weinhold P, et al: A prospective study of tardive dyskinesia development: preliminary results. J Clin Psychopharm 2:345–349, 1982

Schooler N, Kane J: Research diagnoses for tardive dyskinesia (RD-TD). Arch Gen Psychiatry 39:486–487, 1982

3

Early Depressive Signs in Patients with Tardive Dyskinesia

Murray Alpert, Ph.D.
Michael Rush, Ph.D.

3

Early Depressive Signs in Patients with Tardive Dyskinesia

Other chapters in this volume review the mounting evidence for an association between affective illness, especially depression, and tardive dyskinesia (TD). While a number of observations converge on an association between depression and TD, a causal path underlying these observations has not been established because the depression could be a consequence of the mechanisms that produce the TD, or could even result when patients become aware they have an uncontrollable, disfiguring illness. The present study was undertaken to determine whether there was evidence for the existence of depression prior to the development of the TD. To approach this question we undertook a retrospective review of the admission charts of similar groups of patients with and without TD. We appreciate the many problems of interpretation of data from a retrospective chart review but felt that useful although not definitive information might be acquired in a shorter time than would be required for a prospective study.

Method

In a survey of 404 inpatients at the Manhattan Psychiatric Center, 133 patients were found to have TD as judged by two scores of at least two (mild) on the Abnormal Involuntary Movement Scale

(AIMS) (Guy 1974), with at least one of the two ratings in the mouth area (either 2, Lips; 3, Jaw; or 4, Tongue). This criterion with its emphasis on mouth is a bit more stringent than the Research Diagnostic Criteria (RDC) for TD (Kane and Schooler 1981). From the TD group, 11 patients were found who could be matched with eight non-TD controls (no AIMS score above a one) on the following criteria: present in the hospital and still meeting the AIMS criteria six months after the first examination; TD subjects and their controls were matched for current age (within five years); and age at first admission (within five years); and sex; also, we required that the charts from the patients' first admission had to be available. These strict inclusion criteria greatly restricted the number of eligible patients. All appropriate patients were included. In three cases we were able to match two TD patients to one control yielding a total of 11 in the TD group and eight in the control group. In Table 1 the sex, age, and age at first admission are presented for each subject.

Each chart was reviewed by one of us without knowledge as to whether the patient eventually developed TD, and was given a retrospective chart diagnosis according to Research Diagnostic Criteria (Spitzer and Endicott 1980). In addition, each patient was examined for current RDC diagnosis. This examination was, of course, not blind as to TD status. The three diagnoses (admission, retrospective chart, and current RDC) are also noted in Table 1.

The presence of clinically relevant signs and symptoms at the time of the first admission, as recorded in the patients' charts, were rated independently by two raters blind as to TD status. The raters used a checklist consisting of 46 items that are frequently noted in charts. The items were divided into areas such as formal thought disorder, thought content, mood and affect, motor disturbance, and more. The raters were instructed to make a check each time one of the items on the list was mentioned in the chart. Cognate terms used in the charts were to be noted but the raters were instructed to interpret the comments as little as possible. The raters practiced together on extra charts until adequate reliability was achieved. The interrater reliability (product moment correlation) for the two raters independently evaluating the 19 study

Table 1 Overview of Patients in Retrospective Review

		Sex	Age	Age at Last Admission	Admission Diagnosis	RDC Chart Diagnosis	Current RDC Diagnosis
1	TD	M	60	20	Dementia Praecox Paranoid (DP-P)	Tourette Syndrome	Other Psychiatric Diagnosis (Tourette Syndrome)
1	TD	M	60	20	DP-P	Bipolar I	Bipolar I
1	C	M	63	20	DP-P	Schiz./Disorgan.	Schiz./Disorgan.
2	TD	F	66	37	Alcohol Psychosis/ Paranoid	Alcohol Psychosis	Organic Brain Syndrome
2	C	F	62	32	DP-P	Schiz./Paranoid	Schiz.-Aff./Schiz.
3	TD	M	25	22	Schiz./C.U.T.	Bipolar I	Bipolar I
3	C	M	24	19	Schiz./CAT.	Schiz./Mixed	Schiz.-Aff./Schiz.
4	TD	F	60	37	DP-P	Bipolar I	Bipolar I
4	TD	F	61	39	DP-Mixed	Bipolar I	Bipolar I
4	C	F	59	36	DP-P	Schiz./Paranoid	Schiz./Paranoid
5	TD	M	61	27	DP-P	Substance Abuse-Alcohol	Major Affective Disorder/Depr.
5	C	M	60	22	DP-CAT.	Schiz.-Aff./Schiz.	Schiz./Residual
6	TD	F	65	17	DP-CAT.	Bipolar I	Schiz.-Aff./Manic
6	TD	F	70	22	DP-P	Major Depr. Dis./ Depressed	Major Depressive Disorder/Depressed
6	C	F	70	22	DP-CAT.	Schiz./CAT.	Schiz./Undifferentiated
7	TD	M	36	12	Childhood Schiz.	(Attention Deficit Disorder/Childhood)	Anti-Social Personality Disorder/ Paranoid Personality
7	C	M	38	18	Schiz./Mixed	Schiz./Undiff.	Schiz./Undiff.
8	TD	F	69	38	DP-P	Bipolar I	Bipolar I
8	C	F	67	36	DP-P	Schiz./Paranoid	Schiz./Paranoid

NOTE. Mean ± SD age of TD patients at admission, 26.4 ± 9.67 years; mean ± SD age of controls at admission, 25.6 ± 7.7 years. CAT. = catatonic; C.U.T. = chronic undifferentiated type.

charts was $r = .91$ ($p < .01$). Presence of symptoms at first admission and frequencies over the course of hospitalization were converted into rates per hundred lines of notation to control for differences in chart size. Where the information was available, the ratings were kept separate for periods prior to the administration of neuroleptic drugs (many of our patients had been in the hospital for years prior to the introduction of chlorpromazine). For these patients, the ratings were also kept separate for the first several six-month periods of their exposure to neuroleptics.

RESULTS

Table 1 shows that the match for current age and age at admission is good except for dyad no. 7, where the TD patient's first admission was at age 12 and the control's was at age 18. In practically every instance the admission diagnosis was dementia praecox or schizophrenia. The blind chart rediagnosis tended to change for the TD group, in seven cases to affective disorder. This tendency did not appear in the control group. In point of fact, there was no TD patient whose chart qualified for RDC criteria for schizophrenia (one was schizo-affective/mania). The χ^2 value for change in rediagnosis for each group was highly significant ($p < .001$). In other cohorts we have certainly seen TD patients with schizophrenia and we are surprised at the uniformity of nonschizophrenic diagnoses in the TD group. However, our findings are consistent with the suggestion that patients with affective disorders or signs of brain damage are much more likely to appear in the dyskinetic population than would be expected from their representation in the population exposed to neuroleptic drugs.

Some of the results from the ratings of total signs and symptoms on first admission are presented in Figure 1. Here it can be seen that the group that years later developed TD showed less pathology on first admission to the hospital when compared with the non-TD controls ($t = 2.1$, $p < .05$). However, despite less overall pathology, this group had higher scores for signs and symptoms in the mood area ($t = 1.8$, $p < .05$). It is interesting that these chart notations were made, for 15 of the 19 subjects, while the patients were not receiving neuroleptic drugs. Also included in Figure 1 is a comparison of the two groups for psychomotor retardation. Contrary to the other indicators of depression, this indicator was higher in the group that did not later develop TD ($t = 2.8$, $p < .01$). Six of the eight controls but only two of the 11 TD subjects were rated positively on this symptom at first admission. While this finding is open to various interpretations, it may suggest that retardation is found frequently in schizophrenics who are likely to become chronic.

We attempted to analyze the results from the chart review of signs and symptoms to determine if the patients who eventually developed TD showed a different response on first exposure to neuroleptics than did those who did not develop TD, despite similar exposure. We could not use all of our study subjects for this analysis since some subjects were medicated at the time of their first admission. We found that the previously observed differences, wherein the non-TD group showed greater signs and symptoms than did the group that later developed TD, were still

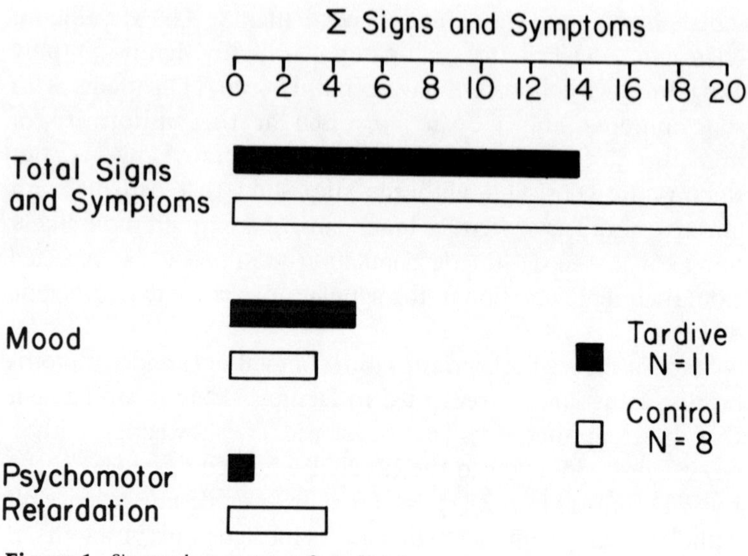

Figure 1 Signs and symptoms at first admission.

discernible but no longer statistically reliable although the reverse was true for scores in the mood area. When medicated, the two groups became more similar as to their overall level of pathology.

It is our impression from inspection of several of the cases that patients in the TD group showed a lesser therapeutic response to neuroleptic medication than did the others. It cannot be stated with confidence that we are observing real differences in response to treatment in the two groups, or whether any difference in treatment response is simply an artifact of difference in the baseline from which the two groups began treatment. We mention the observation because of the clinical implications. We also examined the data from the chart review for evidence that the two groups differed in their tendency to show extrapyramidal side effects when the patients were first exposed to neuroleptic drugs. The information in the charts was not adequate to test for a possible difference in this area.

DISCUSSION

Through an extensive examination of first admission summaries and subsequent chart data, plus criteria-based rediagnosis of old charts, it appears that an increased rate of depression preceded the development of the TD. An interesting and inexplicable aspect of our results is the suggestion that schizophrenics may be resistant to the development of TD. Although based on a small sample, our observations implicating a role for depression are consistent with other findings and suggest a causal path between depression and TD. If these findings can be replicated they have implications for treatment, suggesting caution when placing nonschizophrenic patients, especially those with affective disorders, on neuroleptic drugs for extended periods. The results imply that the risks for such patients are increased and the potential benefits are reduced since they appear to respond less well than the controls to the neuroleptic treatment.

If there is a causal path between depression and TD it is not clear what mechanism underlies this path. Perhaps Sulser's (1978) suggestion that the pharmacodynamic mechanism underlying antidepressant action is mediated via a reduction in the sensitivity of brain noradrenergic receptors may be taken to suggest that depressives tend more easily than others to show increase in catecholamine receptors. An increase in the sensitivity of dopamine receptors has been implicated in the pathophysiology of TD, and patient groups more prone to increased receptor sensitivity may be at greater risk for TD when exposed to neuroleptics. It has long been recognized that the hypothesis of dopamine supersensitivity could not be a complete explanation for the pathogenesis of TD since upregulation of dopamine receptors may be assumed to occur in all patients exposed to neuroleptics, while only some patients go on to develop TD. Some mechanism in addition to receptor supersensitivity is required to explain the great individual differences in vulnerability to TD. In light of Sulser's hypothesis, the possible implication of a defect in receptor adjustment mechanisms, suggested by the vulnerability of depressed patients, seems intuitively reasonable.

References

Guy W: ECDEU Assessment Manual for Psychopharmacology (revised 1976). Washington, DC, US Public Health Service, 1976, pp 534–537

Schooler N, Kane JM: Research diagnoses for tardive dyskinesia (RD-TD). Arch Gen Psychiatry 39:486–487, 1982

Spitzer R, Endicott J: Schedule for affective disorders and schizophrenia (SADS), 3rd ed, updated. New York, New York State Psychiatric Institute, Biometrics Research, 1980

Sulser F: Functional aspects of the norepinephrine receptor-coupled adenylate cyclase system in the limbic forebrain and its modification by drugs which precipitate or alleviate depression: molecular approaches to an understanding of affective disorders. Pharmakopsychiatry Neuropsychopharmakology 11:43–52, 1978

4

Biological Markers and Treatment of Affective Disorder Patients with Tardive Dyskinesia

Alan Rosenbaum, M.D.

4

Biological Markers and Treatment of Affective Disorder Patients with Tardive Dyskinesia

Tardive dyskinesia (TD) is a buccal-lingual masticatory triad associated frequently with abnormal movements of the extremities, and occasionally of the trunk. Antipsychotic drugs which block dopamine appear to be associated with the hypersensitivity phenomenon that is theoretically related to the onset of TD (American College of Neuropsychopharmacology 1973).

In the mid-1970s the increased susceptibility of primary affective disorders to the development of TD was first suggested (Alpert et al. 1976; Davis et al. 1976; Rosenbaum et al. 1977). Of the initial case reports, some of the patients presented with delusional and others with anxious depressions (Rosenbaum et al. 1980a; Rosenbaum et al. 1977; Rosenbaum et al. 1980b). In recent years, more evidence has accumulated showing the increased susceptibility of patients with affective disorders to the development of TD (Kane et al. 1980; Casey 1983; Kane et al. 1983; Wolf et al. 1983).

Further, endocrine testing done in 18 consecutive patients, most of whom had a major depressive disorder (MDD) revealed elevation of urinary free cortisol in 72 percent of these patients. Values ranged from 81 to 630 μg/24 hours. The mean was 198 μg/24 hours versus 66 μg/24 hours for controls ($p < 0.01$, one-tailed Student's *t*-test). Thyroid-stimulating hormone (TSH) levels of these subjects were near zero (Rosenbaum et al. 1979a).

Neuroendocrine testing as well as sleep studies have proven useful as biological markers for depression (Carroll et al. 1976; Carroll et al. 1981; Rosenbaum 1983). The dexamethasone suppression test (DST) is the most established of these tests. Cortisol values above 5 μg at 8:00 A.M., 4:00 P.M. and/or 11:00 P.M. appear as valuable markers when nutritional state and drug effects are taken into account. The thyrotropin-releasing hormone (TRH) test for TSH seems to enhance the sensitivity of neuroendocrine testing for affective disorders, as do sleep studies (Asnis et al. 1983; Targum 1983). A major metabolite of norepinephrine, 3-methoxy-4-hydroxyphenylglycol (MHPG), has been used to subtype depressive disorders (Rosenbaum et al. 1983; Schatzberg et al. 1980; Schatzberg et al. 1981; Schildkraut et al. 1981.)

In previous publications my colleagues and I reported a positive therapeutic effect on TD and the depression with a small-dose antipsychotic–tricyclic antidepressant combination, a lithium–tricyclic combination, and electroconvulsive therapy (ECT) with a lithium–tricyclic combination (Rosenbaum et al. 1977; Rosenbaum et al. 1980a; Rosenbaum et al. 1980b).

To confirm the diagnosis and elucidate the type of depressive disorder we undertook the following study.

METHODS

Patients 45 to 75 years of age with a diagnosis of TD as determined by a psychiatrist and a neurologist were enrolled in the study if they had a TD of at least six-month's duration. Patients had to have a diagnosis of major depressive disorder or manic-depressive disorder (depressed type). All patients were free of psychotropic drugs for a minimum of seven days prior to neuroendocrine, MHPG collections, and sleep studies.

A history was taken and all patients were given a physical examination. Those with a significant medical disorder were excluded from the study. Patients had a Hamilton Depression Rating Scale (HDRS) and a Family History Research Diagnostic Criteria interview done.

Polysomnography (rapid eye movement [REM] latency) of less

than 60 minutes was considered abnormal; a 1-mg DST (with a cutoff of 5 μg/dl at 8:00 A.M., 4:00 P.M., and 11:00 P.M., and a TRH stimulation test for TSH (200 μU of TRH was injected intravenously and a blood sample was obtained after 30 minutes; a change of <5 μU/ml was interpreted as abnormal) were done on all patients. Two 24-hour urine collections for MHPG were done and averaged.

RESULTS

Five patients who fit criteria for TD and MDD enrolled in the study. HDRS scores ranged from 13 to 28 with a mean ± SD of 19.2 ± 6.3.

Four of five patients had positive DST results. All had cortisol values >8 μg/dl at one time period. Two had values $>$ 20 μg/dl at a time period. The fifth patient had a markedly decreased REM latency time, as did three of the five patients overall. All three had REM latencies of 25 minutes or less.

TRH stimulation for TSH was within normal limits for all five patients. MHPG levels, however, showed marked fluctuation. One patient had persistently low levels (mean ± SD, 1,150 μg/24 hours) and three averaged 1,900 μg/24 hours or higher.

DISCUSSION

A number of MDD patients present with anxiety and/or delusions. This appears to be the main reason for the use of phenothiazines. Yet no studies show that antipsychotic drugs alone are useful for the treatment of anxious or delusional depressions.

In previous publications my colleagues and I have shown that there are different subtypes of depressive disorders. The intermediate and high MHPG values ($>$1,950 and $>$2,500 μg/24 hours, respectively) seen in most of our patients do not respond well to standard doses of tricyclic and tetracyclic treatment (Rosenbaum et al. 1980c; Schatzberg et al. 1980; Schatzberg et al. 1981; Schildkraut et al. 1981).

Apparently, these patients already have a high output of

norepinephrine as measured by MHPG. Therefore, the addition of an antidepressant alone to increase norepinephrine would not seem reasonable and, as our previous publications have shown, does not work well. The patients appear anxious, have a high output of cortisol, and are highly DST positive (Jimerson et al. 1983; Rosenbaum et al. 1983).

In a recent publication, Schatzberg et al. have shown delusional depressions to be highly DST positive (>15 μg/dl). Other recent publications have shown manic patients (Krishman et al. 1983), as well as those with atypical psychoses but not those with schizophrenia, to be dexamethasone positive (Arana et al. 1983).

Further studies have shown a positive relationship between dexamethasone positive and shortened REM latency depressions (Asnis et al. 1983). In Asnis' study four of five patients were nonsuppressors to dexamethasone and the fifth had a shortened REM latency. Three of the five patients had agitated depressions, one had a bipolar II disorder, and the fifth presented with pain, decreased energy, decreased interest, and sleep disturbance. Three of the five denied dysphoria but had no interest or energy. All five had been treated with phenothiazines. The TRH stimulation test for TSH was not useful in this small sample of patients but has been in other samples I have seen.

To treat this type of resistant depression in the past, I have used a combination of lithium and a tricyclic antidepressant (Rosenbaum et al. 1977; Rosenbaum et al. 1980a; Rosenbaum et al. 1980b). Approximately 50 percent of patients responded with a diminution of both depression and dyskinesia (11 of 19 showed moderate or marked improvement). The dyskinesia appeared to subside slowly over the ensuing months. Dystonic dyskinesias appeared to respond much more dramatically to treatment than the depressed, nondystonic dyskinesias.

In the present study, two of the patients were not able to tolerate lithium and imipramine or lithium alone because of tremor. One patient receiving imipramine alone cycled up and down and couldn't tolerate lithium because of psoriasis. The patient with bipolar II disorder showed marked organicity but improved enough on the lithium and imipramine to live at home and attend a day care center. The fifth, a 70-year-old lawyer, was able to return to the practice of law on the same medication.

ECT also relieves the depression and dyskinesia in some cases (Rosenbaum et al. 1980b), but patients appear to relapse rapidly unless maintenance medication is used. (In my experience, the longest period before relapse was two months.) One patient who had ECT and was followed for two months became depressed, dyskinetic, and DST positive at the same time.

Although antidepressants have anticholinergic action, and whereas some authors have implicated centrally acting anticholinergic drugs as a causative factor in TD, this has not been proven (Gardos and Cole 1983).

For TD associated with schizophrenia, lecithin (Gelenberg et al. 1982) and choline can be helpful. However, they have been shown to worsen the depression in selected patients with affective disorders (Tamminga et al. 1976). L-Dopa desensitization (Alpert and Friedhoff 1982), which also appears useful for TD, does not treat depression but may prove useful along with lithium and a tricyclic. Reserpine, which can worsen depression, has been reported to worsen dyskinesias (Donatelli et al. 1983), although it is effective for schizophrenia-related TD.

Since the biological markers appear as a useful tool to differentiate schizophrenia from affective disease, I feel that lithium and a tricyclic antidepressant are worth trying for resistant, agitated depression and delusional depressions. Recent studies have confirmed this combination for resistant (Rosenbaum et al. 1979b; de Montigny et al. 1983; Heninger et al. 1983) and delusional depressions (Price et al. 1983). Moreover, lithium, which is a mood stabilizing drug, has been shown to reduce the sum of urinary outputs of dopamine and its major metabolites. This fact may be important in treating depression and TDs (Linnoila et al. 1983). ECT can be used, if needed, followed by maintenance drug therapy. Small dose phenothiazines can be used in combination with a tricyclic antidepressant (Spiker et al. 1982).

For those patients who are DST positive and who are manic or have atypical psychoses, a trial of lithium with an antipsychotic is recommended. Carbamazepine also is sometimes helpful (Folks et al. 1982). In my experience, this treatment allows for a far smaller dose of antipsychotic drug than is normally used, and one is sometimes able to avoid their use entirely.

One difficulty concerning use of the biological markers is that many antipsychotic drugs, especially those with significant anticholinergic action, suppress the cortisols in the DST and make it look negative. Benzodiazepines can suppress the test also.

Further, lithium should not be added to an antipsychotic drug, especially if the patient has been receiving the antipsychotic drug for a long time and is in a depression. This appears to make the depression and dyskinesia worse. Some patients may develop an organic brain syndrome. A drug-free period of three weeks is usually indicated before using lithium (Rosenbaum 1978). (The role of lithium in schizophrenia and TD is discussed in the following chapter.)

For patients who have remained nonresponsive, preliminary findings indicate that a small dose of haloperidol (0.25 to 1.0 mg) added to lithium and a tricyclic is sometimes helpful in retarded depressions. Also, carbamazepine occasionally helps in agitated depressions.

CONCLUSION

Biological markers are useful for patients with MDD and TD. While many of these patients present with nondysphoric depressions, they do have decreased energy and interest and increased anxiety associated with sleep disturbance. The biological markers can confirm the diagnosis. Many patients fall into a group that are nonresponders to typical tricyclic or tetracyclic treatment. About 50 percent will respond to a combination of lithium and a tricyclic antidepressant. Then dyskinesia is usually slow to respond (two to four months) and does not correlate with improvement in the depression.

References

Alpert M, Diamond F, Friedhoff AJ: Tremographic studies in tardive dyskinesia. Psychopharmacol Bull 12:5–7, 1976

Alpert M, Friedhoff AJ: A treatment approach directed toward decreasing receptor sensitivity, in Tardive Dyskinesia and Related Involuntary Movement Disorders: The Long-Term Effects of Antipsychotic Drugs. Edited by DeVeaugh-Geiss J. Boston, John Wright–PSG, 1982

American College of Neuropsychopharmacology–Food and Drug Administration Task Force: Neurologic syndromes associated with antipsychotic-drug use. N Engl J Med 289:20–23, 1973

Arana GW, Barreira PJ, Cohen BM, et al: The dexamethasone suppression test in psychotic disorders. Am J Psychiatry 140:1521–1523, 1983

Asnis GM, Halbreich U, Sachar EJ: Plasma cortisol secretion and REM period latency in adult endogenous depression. Am J Psychiatry 140:750–753, 1983

Carroll BJ, Curtis GC, Davies BM, et al: Urinary free cortisol excretion in depression. Psychol Med 6:43–50, 1976

Carroll BJ, Feinberg M, Greden JF, et al: A specific laboratory test for the diagnosis of melancholia: standardization, validation and clinical utility. Arch Gen Psychiatry 38:15–22, 1981

Casey DE: Tardive dyskinesia and affective disorders. Paper presented at the 136th Annual Meeting of the American Psychiatric Association. New York, May 1983 (Chapter 1 of this monograph)

Davis KL, Berger PA, Hollister LE: Tardive dyskinesia and depressive illness. Psychopharmacology Communications 2:125–130, 1976

de Montigny C, Cournoyer G, Morissette R, et al: Lithium carbonate addition in tricyclic antidepressant-resistant unipolar depression: correlations with the neurobiologic actions of tricyclic antidepressant drugs and lithium ion on the serotonin system. Arch Gen Psychiatry 40:1327–1334, 1983

Donatelli A, Geisen L, Feuer E: Case report of adverse effect of Reserpine on tardive dyskinesia. Am J Psychiatry 140:239–240, 1983

Folks DG, King LD, Dowdy SB, et al: Carbamazepine treatment of selected affectively disordered inpatients. Am J Psychiatry 139:115–117, 1982

Gardos G, Cole JD: Tardive dyskinesia and anticholinergic drugs. Am J Psychiatry 140:200–202, 1983

Gelenberg AJ, Wojcik JD, Growdon JH, et al: Lecithin for the treatment of tardive dyskinesia: preliminary results from a double-blind study, in Tardive Dyskinesia and Related Involuntary Movement Disorders: The Long-Term Effects of Antipsychotic Drugs. Edited by DeVeaugh-Geiss J. Boston, John Wright–PSG, 1982

Heninger GR, Charney DS, Sternberg DE: Lithium carbonate augmentation of antidepressant treatment: an effective prescription for treatment-refractory depression. Arch Gen Psychiatry 40:1335–1342, 1983

Jimerson DC, Insel TR, Reus VI, et al: Increased plasma MHPG in dexamethasone-resistant depressed patients. Arch Gen Psychiatry 40:173–176, 1983

Kane J, Struve FA, Weinhold P, et al: Strategy for the study of patients at high risk for tardive dyskinesia. Am J Psychiatry 137:1265–1267, 1980

Kane J, Woerner M, Weinhold P, et al: Incidence and severity of tardive dyskinesia in affective illness. Paper presented at the 136th Annual Meeting of the American Psychiatric Association. New York, May 1983 (Chapter 2 of this monograph)

Krishman RR, Maltbie AA, Davidson JRT: Abnormal cortisol suppression in bipolar patients with simultaneous manic and depressive symptoms. Am J Psychiatry 140:203–205, 1983

Linnoila M, Karoum F, Potter WZ: Effects of antidepressant treatments on dopamine turnover in depressed patients. Arch Gen Psychiatry 40:1015–1017, 1983

Price LH, Conwell Y, Nelson JC: Lithium augmentation of combined neuroleptic-tricyclic treatment in delusional depression. Am J Psychiatry 140:318–322, 1983

Rosenbaum AH: Tardive dyskinesia and pharmacotherapy (ltr to ed). Am J Psychiatry 135:506, 1978

Rosenbaum AH: The laboratory and the practicing clinical psychiatrist, in Human Disease (A.O. Beckman Conference). Winston-Salem, North Carolina, AACC Publications, 1983 (in press)

Rosenbaum AH, Maruta T, Duane DD, et al: Tardive dyskinesia in depressed patients: successful therapy with antidepressants and lithium. Psychosomatics 21:715–719, 1980

Rosenbaum AH, Maruta T, Jiang N-S, et al: Endocrine testing in tardive dyskinesias: preliminary report. Am J Psychiatry 136:102–103, 1979

Rosenbaum AH, Maruta T, Richelson E: Drugs that alter mood, Part II: lithium. Mayo Clin Proc 54:401–407, 1979

Rosenbaum AH, Maruta T, Schatzberg AF, et al: Toward a biochemical classification of depressive disorders, VII: Urinary free cortisol and urinary MHPG in depressions. Am J Psychiatry 140:314–318, 1983

Rosenbaum AH, Niven RG, Hanson NP, et al: Tardive dyskinesia: relationship with a primary affective disorder. Diseases of the Nervous System 38:423–427, 1977

Rosenbaum AH, O'Connor MK, Duane DD, et al: Treatment of tardive dyskinesia in an agitated, depressed patient. Psychosomatics 21:765–766, 1980

Rosenbaum AH, Schatzberg AF, Maruta T, et al: MHPG as a predictor of antidepressant response to imipramine and maprotiline. Am J Psychiatry 137:1090–1092, 1980

Schatzberg AF, Orsulak PJ, Rosenbaum AH, et al: Toward a biochemical classification of depressive disorders, IV: pretreatment urinary MHPG levels as predictors of antidepressant response to imipramine. Commun Psychopharmacol 4:441–445, 1980

Schatzberg AF, Rosenbaum AH, Orsulak PJ, et al: Toward a biochemical classification of depressive disorders, III: pretreatment urinary MHPG levels as predictors of response to treatment with maprotiline. Psychopharmacology (Berlin) 75:34–38, 1981

Schatzberg AF, Rothchild AJ, Stahl J, et al: The dexamethasone suppression test: identification of subtypes of depression. Am J Psychiatry 140:88–91, 1983

Schildkraut JJ, Orsulak PJ, Schatzberg AF, et al: Possible pathophysiological mechanism in subtypes of unipolar depressive disorders based on differences in urinary MHPG levels. Psychopharmacol Bull 17:90–91, 1981

Spiker DG, Rossi AJ, Cofsky JE, et al: Drug therapy for delusional depressives, in Syllabus and Proceedings in Summary Form: the 135th Annual Meeting of the American Psychiatric Association. Washington, DC, American Psychiatric Association, 1982

Tamminga C, Smith RC, Chang S, et al: Depression associated with oral choline (ltr to ed). Lancet 2:905, 1976

Targum SD: The application of serial neuroendocrine challenge studies in the management of depressive disorder. Biol Psychiatry 18:3–19, 1983

Wolf ME, Chevesich J, Lehrer E, et al: The clinical association of tardive dyskinesia and drug induced Parkinsonism. Biol Psychiatry 18:1181–1188, 1983

5

Lithium Carbonate in Tardive Dyskinesia and Schizophrenia

Jonathan O. Cole, M.D.
George Gardos, M.D.
Robert M. Rapkin, M.D.
Joel Gelernter, M.D.
David Haskell, M.D.
Patricia Moore, R.N., M.P.H.
Susan Schniebolk, B.A.
Michael Bird, A.B.

5

Lithium Carbonate in Tardive Dyskinesia and Schizophrenia

Lithium carbonate has long been recognized as an effective treatment for patients with recurring affective disorders, both bipolar and unipolar. Lithium's role in other psychiatric conditions is less clear, though it is sometimes helpful in patients with mood lability or with impulsive anger. All in all, lithium has reasonable credentials as an antipsychotic, at least antimanic, drug. All currently available antipsychotic drugs appear to be able to produce tardive dyskinesia and often fail to produce full remissions in schizophrenic patients. Hence, a drug that can be used to effectively treat schizophrenics, that is not a dopamine blocking agent, and that is free of the danger of tardive dyskinesia is urgently needed. A drug that could partially replace antipsychotics in patients who had developed tardive dyskinesia would be useful, especially if it also ameliorated the dyskinesia. Even a drug that could be added to standard antipsychotics to further benefit patients only partially improved on antipsychotics alone would be helpful.

In the years since clozapine was removed from clinical use because of its association with agranulocytosis, no new antischizophrenic drug has emerged with any of the desirable properties noted above. It is therefore worthwhile to reassess the evidence that an old drug, lithium carbonate, is a candidate for one or more of the roles described above. We completed a small study with these issues in mind. However, the literature review will be presented first and the study subsequently.

Should Lithium Help Tardive Dyskinesia?

Apparently the first mention of lithium carbonate used for a movement disorder in the literature was a letter by Dalen (1973), who claimed that a 65-year-old woman with severe tardive dyskinesia (TD) responded very well "as soon as an adequate blood level of lithium was reached." He also treated six Huntington's chorea patients with lithium (range, 0.7–1.5 mEq/liter) and found a "striking reduction" in hyperkinetic movements in three of the six. In another anecdotal account, Simpson (1973) reported that "TD disappeared in three manic patients when they were switched from neuroleptics to lithium therapy." Improvement was also seen in nonmanic patients' TD as well when they were switched to lithium. In another small trial, Prange et al. (1973) treated two TD patients with increasing doses of lithium in a double-blind study. Marked dose-related improvement was seen, with patients relapsing when placebo was substituted for lithium. Lithium levels were not reported. Pickar and Davies (1978) described a case of TD in a 23-year-old woman who was treated with lithium. They reported that there was some improvement with a level between 0.4 and 0.6 mEq/liter, but deterioration with a level between 0.6 and 1.0 mEq/liter. This patient was later treated by one of us (J.C.). We were unable to reproduce the earlier differential effect of high and low lithium levels. Reda et al. (1975) reported an open trial of lithium in the treatment of TD in six patients (ages 46–67 years) with alternating two-week lithium/no lithium/lithium periods. Blood levels of lithium were adjusted to lie at 0.7–1.0 mEq/liter. Previous medications were continued throughout the trial. There was a statistically significant improvement while the patients were receiving lithium, but it was small, generally in the range of 15 to 20 percent.

In a larger trial with double-blind crossover design, Gerlach et al. (1975) compared lithium with placebo in TD. Fifteen patients (12 receiving antipsychotic medications) were given three-week trials, keeping lithium levels between 0.8 and 1.2 mEq/liter. Their other medications were not changed as they entered the trial. The dyskinesia improved moderately (average reduction in score, 25 percent) when the subjects were receiving lithium. Best improvement was seen at a serum lithium level of 0.8 mEq/liter; there was a therapeutic window effect with patients with higher serum levels showing some, but not maximal, improvement. Concurrent antipsychotic therapy had no effect on lithium response. Jus et al. (1978) did a larger ($N = 23$) double-blind crossover study of deanol, lithium, and placebo in chronic schizophrenics with TD (ages, 39–60 years). The patients' antipsychotic medications were continued through the trial. Each medication was administered for eight weeks with washout periods between trials. For the lithium section of the trial, low doses of the drug were used (mean level, 350 mg), and plasma levels were 0.7–0.9 mEq/liter. No statistically significant results accrued, but two patients deteriorated when on lithium, and five patients improved. In the cases where there was improvement, it persisted for one to two months after the lithium had been discontinued. Simpson et al. (1976) did a double-blind study of lithium in TD with a result that he interpreted as negative. Antipsychotic medication was withdrawn over six weeks, gradually in some patients and abruptly in others. Then, after at least four weeks on placebo only, the double-blind crossover study was begun. Study periods were six weeks each for lithium (range, 0.6–1.0 mEq/liter; mean level, 0.71 mEq/liter) and placebo. Five of the original 16 patients could not tolerate the neuroleptic withdrawal and relapsed. In the 10 patients who finished the trial (mean age, 72 years), there was no significant change in dyskinetic symptoms.

Mackay et al. (1980) also came up with negative results in a placebo-controlled double-blind study of 11 neuroleptic-maintained TD patients. Serum lithium levels were held between 0.8–1.3 mEq/liter. No consistent change in TD or psychiatric state was associated with lithium treatment. Ereshefsky et al. (1979) present a complex case of a woman with bipolar disorder who had manifested TD since she was shifted from antipsychotics to lithium six years earlier. During an admission which began with confusion, ataxia, and lithium toxicity but with no evidence of dyskinesia, the patient developed both mania and marked dyskinesia as her toxicity cleared. Both conditions ameliorated in another 10 days. The authors assert that red blood cell/plasma lithium ratios correlated better with dyskinesia suppression than did plasma levels alone.

There are reports of lithium use for related movement disorders as well. Following the Dalen report cited earlier, Aminoff and Marshall (1974) studied nine Huntington's chorea patients in a double-blind trial of lithium carbonate. Other medications were not changed; six patients were receiving antipsychotics. "There was no improvement in the abnormal movements" or in other measures; all patients were unchanged or worse. Levels were in the range of 0.6–1.5 mEq/liter. Leonard et al. (1974) studied lithium, lithium plus haloperidol, haloperidol, and placebo in a double-blind trial, also for Huntington's chorea. Each treatment was used for three weeks. Lithium levels were 0.8–1.2 mEq/liter. Abnormal movements were not significantly affected by *any* treatment. Other symptoms (anger and irritability) were helped slightly by lithium, moderately by haloperidol, and most by the two together. Hamra et al. (1983) gave lithium to a patient with cyclothymic disorder and chronic tic disorder, the latter present for five years. The tics gradually improved and then disappeared over the course of two months. (This suggests that in some of the earlier studies lithium use may not have been continued long enough.)

Some investigators have found lithium to have a negative effect in treatment of movement disorders. Beitman (1978) offered a case report in which a 56-year-old woman's dyskinesia was apparently reinduced by lithium after four years of quiescence; her dyskinesia was suppressed by trihexyphenidyl. Crews and Carpenter (1977) published a single case report of a 46-year-old woman in which the time course of worsening of TD suggested a relationship to lithium use, but with very high (2 mEq/liter) serum levels of lithium. A confounding factor was the discontinuation of the patient's antipsychotic the week before high-dose lithium was begun.

Several cases have been described in which severe lithium toxicity, generally with concomitant haloperidol medication, led to an organic dementia with the emergence of a persistent TD (Cohen and Cohen 1974). However, a recent review of neurologic sequelae of long-term lithium therapy did not reveal any additional instances of persistent dyskinesia (Donaldson and Cunningham 1983). Reversible neurotoxicity, including dyskinesia, was noted by Prakash et al. (1982).

What can be concluded from this heterogeneous group of studies? There appear to be occasional patients whose TD improves markedly or moderately when lithium is administered. In some cases antipsychotics were concurrently stopped; in other cases it is not stated whether antipsychotics were continued or not. In studies using placebo controls or on-off designs, results are far less impressive. Sometimes a modest 20 to 25 percent decrease in movements is seen; sometimes no drug-placebo difference is found. There is a suggestion that lithium serum level may make a difference. Toxic levels can induce (or suppress) dyskinesia. Perhaps lower therapeutic levels (0.4–0.7 mEq/liter) are better than higher levels. Probably older, more chronic patients are less likely to respond. Longer treatment durations (e.g., at least two months) may be needed in some patients for full response to occur.

Does Lithium Help Schizophrenia?

Cade, the originator of lithium therapy in psychiatry, reported in 1949 on the first six schizophrenic patients ever treated with lithium, noting that "although there was no fundamental improvement in any of them, three who were usually restless, noisy, and shouting nonsensical abuse . . . lost their excitement and restlessness and became quiet and amenable for the first time in years. . . . They reverted to their previous state upon cessation of lithium medication" (Cade 1949). Subsequent studies of lithium in schizophrenia can be divided roughly into two groups. Some investigators begin with the presumption that schizoaffective disorder, variously described, may be a variant of bipolar disorder and therefore might be lithium responsive. Other investigators are interested in the response of schizophrenics per se, to lithium. The studies end up overlapping because many schizophrenics show some affective features. In fact, one study (Biederman et al. 1979) defined six clinical subtypes going from manic excitement with delusions or hallucinations to patients without affective symptoms—chronic schizophrenics. The issues, however, are clearer than the diagnostic distinctions may be. Does lithium control only manic symptoms in schizophrenic patients or does it have a broader antipsychotic effect?

As noted, some studies of lithium in schizophrenia have elected to concentrate on patients exhibiting significant affective symptoms. This was the approach of Rapp and Edwards (1977). They developed an original rating scale of 10 items selected to correlate with bipolar affective disorder (e.g., family history of affective illness, good functioning between psychotic episodes, personal warmth); only those patients from a schizophrenia clinic who met at least five of the criteria were eligible for the study. Nine patients were selected for a lithium trial; blood levels were 0.5–0.9 mEq/liter. Eight of the nine patients responded well, apparently on lithium and off antipsychotics. The authors conclude that this demonstrates that lithium-responsive bipolar patients are to be found regularly among schizophrenics, sharing their treatments and potentially deprived of the benefit of more effective ones. Rapp and Edwards did not, however, further test their hypothesis by giving lithium to any of the presumably less "affective" patients in their original sample.

Many other investigators have found the idea of trying lithium in schizoaffective patients seductive. Hussain and Gomersall (1978) reported three case histories in which lithium was given to schizoaffectives refractory to other medications, essentially as a last resort, with excellent results; at least one of the three was also continued on antipsychotics. Brockington et al. (1978) described a small study where lithium or chlorpromazine was given double-blind to "manic schizoaffective" patients. The lithium alone was found to work as well as the chlorpromazine, decreasing both affective and psychotic symptoms. Johnson (1970) evoked good lithium results with 19 manic patients, but poor results with 11 excited schizoaffective patients. Lithium was pushed to the point of side effects and the resulting levels were very high (maxima, 1.00–2.55 mEq/liter), perhaps accounting for the poor responses.

Prien et al. (1972) compared lithium (levels, 0.6–2.0 mEq/liter) and chlorpromazine in a group of 83 newly admitted schizoaffective excited patients. Study medication was continued for three weeks. In about half of the patients ("mildly active"), lithium was as good as chlorpromazine; in the other more disturbed group, chlorpromazine was superior in all areas. However, 59 percent of these lithium patients were dropped from the study in the first 10 days for uncontrollable behavior or side effects. Some of these *might* have responded if they had been able to be sustained on lithium for the full three weeks. Lithium was, again, not found to be specific for affective symptoms.

Biederman et al. (1979) compared haloperidol with and without lithium (plasma levels approximately 1.0 mEq/liter) in a group of 18 "excited schizoaffective" patients for five weeks. Once again the added lithium was found to be of "modest but consistent beneficial effect" for many symptoms, not just those associated with mania. The improvement was slightly more pronounced in those patients who were closer to the schizophrenic than the affective end of the schizoaffective spectrum. The patients receiving lithium and haloperidol were also less likely to develop depressive symptoms than those on haloperidol alone.

Glazer and Sheard (1982) screened a population of 60 outpatients diagnosed as schizophrenic and selected four of those with past history of both affective-type and schizophrenic-type episodes to study. They discontinued their antipsychotics and substituted lithium (levels, 0.45–1.0 mEq/liter). Over the course of 13 months, one patient improved and three relapsed (one of these had discontinued his lithium). This small, uncontrolled study demonstrates that one cannot simplistically replace antipsychotics with lithium in patients with histories of past schizophrenic-like episodes.

Lithium as an adjunct medication has also been shown to be beneficial in chronic schizophrenic patients. Carmen et al. (1981) studied 11 chronic schizophrenic and seven schizoaffective patients, all with schizoid premorbid adjustment and insidious onset of disease. Lithium or placebo was added to patients' standard neuroleptic treatment; they were assigned to lithium/placebo/lithium or placebo/lithium/placebo groups, with each medication administered for four weeks. Lithium levels were 0.75–1.3 mEq/liter. About half of the chronic schizophrenics benefited from the addition of lithium. This was regarded as a primarily "antimanic" effect, but there was an antipsychotic effect as well. Patients with affective symptoms benefited more. It has been suggested that "good-prognosis schizophrenia" and "schizophreniform disorder" might be atypical presentations of bipolar affective disorder rather than variants of schizophrenia (Pope and Lipinski 1978), and, accordingly, Hirschowitz et al. (1980) characterized lithium response in a group of 31 Research Diagnostic Criteria (RDC) schizoaffectives and schizophrenics. They used a lithium trial of only two weeks' duration (less than the expected time course for the full extent of improvement on lithium, but probably enough time to see some response), with blood levels of 1.1–1.4 mEq/liter. Nine of the patients showed a decrease in schizophrenic symptoms, and seven of these nine showed greater than 30 percent improvement. A different seven of the nine responders had DSM-III schizophreniform disorder. Eight of the 10 patients in the group who met McCabe criteria for good-prognosis schizophrenia were among the responders. Nonschizophreniform patients, whether depressed schizoaffective or schizophrenic, did not improve in this trial of lithium given alone.

Lithium was studied in schizophrenic patients by Alexander et al. (1979), Growe et al. (1979), and Small et al. (1975). In the first study, lithium was administered to a group of 13 previously drug-free hospitalized schizophrenic patients for three weeks, with placebo given before and after. Levels of 0.7–1.2 mEq/liter were used. Seven of the 13 patients responded to lithium with a mean improvement in psychosis rating of at least 20 percent. When lithium was withdrawn, four of these seven soon relapsed. The only good predictor of response in the third week was response in the first week. Growe et al. and Small et al. both added lithium to the antipsychotics that their patients were receiving. Growe et al. added lithium or placebo to the treatment regimen of eight chronic inpatients (six schizophrenic, two schizoaffective) who were refractory to antipsychotic treatment, in a double-blind crossover trial using four-week medication periods. Levels of 0.5–1.0 mEq/liter were used. Significant improvement was noted only on a "psychotic excitement" scale. Small et al. added lithium to the previous medications of 22 chronic schizophrenic patients, with lithium levels of 0.6–1.0 mEq/liter. Ten of the 22 patients improved, with decreased psychosis and other global improvements. Lithium responders were significantly older and had been hospitalized for significantly longer.

Finally, Delva et al. (1982) approached the issue from the other direction; they identified six chronic schizophrenic patients who had been receiving both lithium and antipsychotics, and withdrew their lithium. Two of the patients relapsed and required reinstitution of lithium within two weeks, but the other four lasted intact for at least a year. This result was thought to support claims of lithium's efficacy as an antipsychotic in some patients.

The available studies of lithium in either schizoaffective disorder or schizophrenia leave the clinician interested but not entirely satisfied. Except for the study of Prien et al. (1972), the relevant studies all have small samples of patients, and many are either open studies or case reports. One by Johnson (1970) is clearly negative but all the others suggest that lithium, either alone or added to an antipsychotic, often has some beneficial effects in at least some of the patients treated. The studies in mainly nonaffective schizophrenics are almost as positive as those in schizoaffectives, only with the caveat that there is no double-blind controlled study comparing lithium with placebo in chronic schizophrenics who are not receiving antipsychotics. The published evidence is compatible with our informal clinical experience, which suggests that lithium is sometimes helpful when added to antipsychotics in both schizoaffectives and, less commonly, in chronic schizophrenics with agitation or impulsive angry outbursts without obvious affective features. Local clinical experience also suggests that, when properly handled, lithium is a low-risk option in treatment-resistant patients. If the patient does not benefit, the clinical condition is not worsened unless the usual lithium side effects occur.

How Might Lithium Act?

Lithium's mechanism of action is still not well understood. An old idea, fitting nicely into the hyperdopaminergic theory of mania and schizophrenia, is that lithium decreases catecholamine release. The more recent evidence that lithium blocks the neuroleptic-induced dopamine receptor proliferation in the brain (Klawans et al. 1977; Pert et al. 1978; Gallager et al. 1978; Goodnick and Meltzer 1983) is potentially more relevant to a possible effect of lithium in preventing the development of TD. Neither of these phenomena based on laboratory studies helps explain very clearly either lithium's positive effect on schizophrenic symptoms or on TD. Clinical observations are not much more helpful. The observation that lithium sometimes causes parkinsonian cogwheeling as well as the more conventional tremor makes one wonder whether lithium is not really a weak neuroleptic, and raises the fear that it might ultimately produce or aggravate TD. There is also clinical evidence that some patients are slowed by lithium and that lithium has occasional efficacy in reducing impulsive anger or assaultiveness.

The above review leaves the role of lithium in the treatment of schizophrenics with TD uncertain if not doubtful. Lithium may indirectly benefit patients with TD. Through its antimanic effect, lithium may effect symptomatic improvement in patients with affective symptomatology. Alternatively, in neuroleptic-treated patients, effective therapy with lithium may enable the neuroleptic drug to be discontinued.

We conducted a double-blind controlled study that explored these issues. The study had three interlocking aims: (1) to compare lithium carbonate and placebo in patients with TD receiving a steady antipsychotic drug dosage over an eight-week period, looking primarily for changes in dyskinesia; (2) to determine whether the above patients tolerated gradual antipsychotic drug withdrawal better on lithium than on placebo; and (3) to determine whether lithium was superior to placebo in inducing improvement in psychiatric (not dyskinetic) status and whether such improvement was predictable on the basis of prestudy affective features as measured by the Rapp-Edwards (1977) scale.

METHODS

Patient Selection

Patients were inpatients or outpatients with a chart diagnosis of schizophrenia who were receiving stable antipsychotic therapy, under 65 years of age, and without major medical problems or a history of lithium intolerance. Tardive dyskinesia as indicated by at least one "moderate" or two "mild" ratings on the Abnormal Involuntary Movements Scale (Guy 1976) had to have been present for at least three months. Patients with unreliable clinic attendance or poor drug compliance were excluded. All patients gave informed consent for the study.

Settings

Patients were recruited from a variety of settings. These included the Lawrence and Memorial Hospital Clinic in New London, Connecticut (six patients), the Boston Veterans Administration Clinic (seven patients), the McLean Tardive Dyskinesia Clinic (three patients), the Bedford Veterans Administration Hospital (one patient), and the West-Ros-Park Mental Health Center (one patient).

Medication

Double-blind lithium carbonate (300 mg) and matching placebo capsules were provided by Smith, Kline, and French Laboratories. The double-blind status was maintained by having a nonblind clinician at each site provide the blind treating psychiatrist with all serum lithium values. In the case of placebo patients, artificial, predetermined flexible values were provided to maintain the blind. Patients were randomly assigned to lithium or placebo at a ratio of two lithium patients to one placebo patient.

Ratings

Prestudy training in both TD ratings and psychopathology ratings was provided by three of us (J.C., G.G., P.M.), the original trained raters. Reliability was not formally determined, but 20 jointly supervised ratings were done by the raters at each site, either with the three original raters as a group or with one of them during visits to the site. The following ratings were used. (1) The NIMH-PRB Abnormal Involuntary Movements Scale (AIMS) (Guy 1976), which employs global severity ratings of dyskinetic movements in seven body areas on five-point scales. An overall severity rating is also made. (2) The Dyskinesia Rating Scale (DRS) (Simpson et al. 1979), which is a 34-item six-point scale for the rating of discrete abnormal movements (e.g., tongue protrusion, finger counting, stamping movements) that are commonly observed in dyskinetic patients. Items are summed to form cluster scores of choreoathetosis, restlessness, and tremor. (3) The Brief Psychiatric Rating Scale (BPRS) (Overall and Gorham 1962), which is an 18-item psychopathology scale. The BPRS was completed at each rating point. (4) The Global Adjustment Scale (GAS) (Endicott et al. 1976), which provides a single rating of overall adjustment and psychopathology.

Rating Schedule and Study Logistics

For the initial eight-week study, two baseline ratings were obtained before the patients were randomly assigned to lithium or placebo. Ratings were then made every two weeks for eight weeks, antipsychotic dose being held constant. After eight weeks, antipsychotic dosage was reduced by 15 percent to 25 percent every four weeks, and ratings were made every four weeks. After a dosage level of 20 to 25 percent of the original dose had been reached (at about 24 weeks), that dosage was held stable for six months. If the patient was still doing well, antipsychotic drugs were stopped and the patient continued to be followed and rated every four weeks for a year. Lithium or placebo treatment was continued for the duration of the study or until relapse.

Statistical Analysis

An analysis of covariance for multiple time points was used for the first eight-week phase of the study. An endpoint analysis of covariance was also carried out using two baseline ratings and the last rating available on all patients. The latter analysis was chosen because of the highly variable time periods for which patients participated in the study.

RESULTS

Patient recruitment turned out to be a major unanticipated problem. Otherwise suitable patients were often either already receiving lithium or were unwilling to consent to the study. Three years of effort finally yielded only 18 patients who had completed at least eight weeks of the study. At the three-year point we had observed psychotic decompensation in six patients who had been psychiatrically stable for several years prior to the study. The rate of untoward outcomes led to our stopping the study. The reasons for termination by treatment group are listed in Table 1. The administrative terminations all resulted from major staff changes at the New London Clinic. Table 1 also shows that the cohort represented a chronically psychotic, mostly schizophrenic population. The placebo group received lower antipsychotic doses (not statistically significant).

Eight-week Study Phase

On the dyskinesia measures, differences favoring lithium were found. Figure 1 shows that the choreoathetoid cluster of the DRS showed significant improvement on lithium at six and eight weeks, and trends in the same direction at two and four weeks. The Restlessness and Parkinsonism subscales of the DRS did not show significant drug-placebo differences at four and eight weeks, while the AIMS Face score (the sum of items one through four) showed drug-placebo differences at weeks two, four, and eight. Individual AIMS items that showed lithium effect were item two (lips), item three (jaw) at several time points, and item four (tongue) at week eight only. There were no lithium-placebo differences on either clinical status measure: GAS or BPRS.

Extended Study

At week eight, three patients were unwilling to continue on the study because of expressed dissatisfaction with the protocol (e.g., repeated blood tests) or with the subjective effects of the study capsules. All three were found to have been on lithium. When

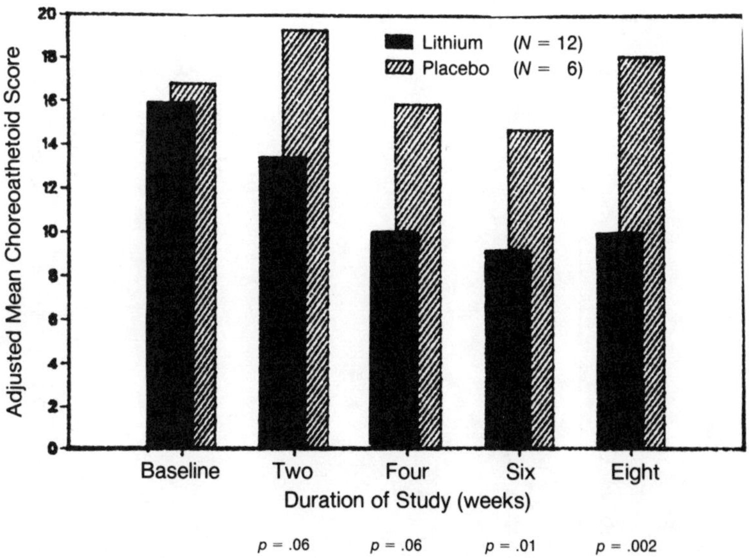

Figure 1 Choreoathetoid scores of patients receiving lithium and placebo. Statistical significance was determined by analysis of covariance (lithium vs placebo) using the baseline score as the covariate.

Table 1 Patient Characteristics

Study Group,	Patient No.	Sex	Age	Duration of Illness (years)	Diagnosis	Medication at Baseline (mg)	Rapp-Edwards Score	Weeks on Study	Reason for Termination
Lithium	33	F	57	30	Schizophrenia/ Paranoid Type	750	0	8	Refused
	34	F	32	10	Schizophrenia/ Undifferentiated Type	400	3	8	Refused
	35	M	39	25	Schizophrenia/ Undifferentiated Type	70	3	8	Lithium side effects
	37	M	40	15	Paranoid Disorder	200	6	10	Refused
	42	M	37	11	Schizophrenia/ Undifferentiated Type	1,150	2	15	Relapse
	56	M	43	28	Mental Retardation	750	0	20	Relapse
	53	F	46	26	Schizo-affective	200	5	23	Lithium side effects
	55	M	59	29	Schizophrenia/ Undifferentiated Type	125	2	27	Administrative
	51	F	38	8	Schizophrenia/ Paranoid Type	465	3	29	Administrative

	06	M	60	28	Schizo-affective	1,000	2	40	Completer
	04	M	58	19	Bipolar Disorder	500	7	48	Suicide attempt
	02	M	54	34	Schizophrenia/ Undifferentiated Type	180	7	60	Completer
Mean ± SD			46.9 ± 10.1	21.9 ± 8.9		482.5 ± 358.4	3.3 ± 2.4	24.7 ± 17.1	
Placebo	54	F	50	13	Schizophrenia/ Undifferentiated Type	1,000	4	23	Administrative
	52	F	36	8	Schizophrenia/ Paranoid Type	100	1	29	Relapse
	07	M	63	18	Schizophrenia/ Undifferentiated Type	120	5	37	Relapse
	05	M	52	30	Schizo-affective	200	4	48	Relapse
	03	M	62	41	Schizophrenia/ Paranoid Type	250	5	52	Relapse
	01	M	59	20	Chronic Anxiety with Depression	320	7	84	Administrative
Mean ± SD			53.7 ± 10.1	21.7 ± 12.0		331.7 ± 337.4	4.3 ± 2.0	45.5 ± 21.8	

changes between week eight and the last study rating are compared for the nine lithium and six placebo patients who continued beyond the eighth week, only one significant difference in the analysis of variance of change scores was found. The placebo patients improved on the choreoathetoid score of the DRS, while the lithium patients worsened, the difference being significant ($F = 10.23$, $p = 0.013$). The AIMS Face and Total scores showed changes in the same direction which did not reach statistical significance. The GAS and BPRS showed weak trends in the same directions, placebo patients being on the average slightly better and lithium patients slightly worse. When initial differences in neuroleptic doses were statistically adjusted for analysis of covariance, the lithium-placebo difference on DRS choreoathetosis just missed significance ($F = 5.51$, $p = .051$). It is necessary to point out that the relapsing patients (four on placebo, two on lithium) were not ratable at the point of actual relapse. Patients often decompensated quite precipitously, and these changes were first observed by community caretakers who appropriately requested immediate intervention with the result that the medication was restarted before a clinic visit could be arranged.

Side Effects

Two patients terminated as a result of lithium side effects: one patient complained of thirst and polyuria with serum levels of 0.7–0.8 mEq/liter and was unwilling to stay on lithium beyond eight weeks. The second patient, a 46-year-old woman, showed thirst, dizziness, ataxia, and a tremor on levels of 0.9–1.0 mEq/liter and discontinued lithium therapy at 23 weeks. Six other patients presented with typical side effects at therapeutic serum levels but tolerated the drug quite well and were willing to continue on the study.

Prediction of Lithium Response

The Rapp-Edwards Scale did not predict clinical improvement on lithium as rated by the BPRS or GAS. The three patients on lithium showing more than 20 percent improvement on the BPRS had Rapp-Edwards scores of six, two, and two. In the lithium group with scores above five that Rapp and Edwards used to select patients for their original study, only one of the four patients improved. None of the improved patients was judged dramatically better by their treating clinicians.

DISCUSSION

The study was beset by recruitment problems prior to its start. We encountered an unexpectedly strong reluctance on the part of otherwise suitable patients to agree to participate. In part this was due to previous negative experiences with lithium, although rarely on the basis of adequate clinical trials with the drug. Resistance to repeated blood tests constituted a further recruitment problem. During the first phase of the study patients did not tolerate lithium well despite the fact that the serum levels were well within the normal range. Of the 12 lithium patients, three refused to continue on lithium beyond eight weeks and two others were terminated from the study because of side effects. These findings support previous suggestions that schizophrenics tolerate the lithium ion less well than affective patients (Shopsin et al. 1970; Prakash et al. 1982). Lithium intolerance may well be a limiting factor in the effective use of lithium in some schizophrenics who might otherwise derive benefit from the drug.

The eight-week phase of the study generally confirms prior studies which had shown or suggested that lithium decreased abnormal movements in patients with TD. The improvement occurred primarily in choreoathetoid movements that are the characteristic abnormalities of TD. Noteworthy as these results are, the changes were more statistically than clinically significant. Observations of striking remission of movements were conspicuously absent. Thus lithium may join the undistinguished ranks of available treatment agents for TD, each of which benefits only a proportion of dyskinetic patients and usually only to a modest degree.

The clinical effects of lithium on psychopathology in this

group of middle-aged, chronically ill, schizophrenic outpatients were not impressive, though occasional patients were judged to be a bit better. Lithium patients were less likely to relapse during antipsychotic dosage withdrawal, though the numbers were too small to be statistically analyzed. There were only two study completers, both in the lithium group. However, there were two other lithium patients in New London who were clinically stable on 20 percent of their neuroleptic dose when the study was discontinued; these patients had decompensated one year previously on placebo while participating in an earlier study. These four apparent lithium successes suggest a degree of prophylactic effectiveness in some chronic schizophrenics. The three lithium patients who decompensated during the extended phase were initially on high neuroleptic doses (500, 750, and 1,150 mg of chlorpromazine daily). The small numbers preclude what would otherwise be an obvious conclusion that lithium is less likely to be effective in schizophrenics requiring high doses of neuroleptics.

The slight worsening of the lithium patients' dyskinesia and the improvement of the placebo patients in the extended portion of the study were confounded by antipsychotic dosage reduction or discontinuation. This raises interesting theoretical possibilities. Perhaps lithium stabilizes dopamine receptors at the level they were at when lithium treatment was instituted. It is thought to have this effect in animals when lithium is given before antipsychotics are added, or when both are initiated simultaneously (Klawans et al. 1977; Pert et al. 1978; Gallager et al. 1978). If lithium stabilized receptors when dopamine receptor proliferation had already occurred, this would result in increased potential for psychosis and movement disorders with discontinuation of the antipsychotics. On the other hand, one would have predicted that neuroleptic withdrawal in the placebo group might cause dyskinesia to increase. Perhaps the lithium-placebo difference is explicable by the larger number of patients with chlorpromazine-equivalent dosages under 400 mg a day in the placebo group (five of six) than in the lithium group (five of 12). Although we know of no data to support the idea, it seems likely that a rebound exacerbation of dyskinesia is more likely to occur in patients on higher initial neuroleptic dosage. There was in fact a correlation (nonsignificant) of .49 between the initial chlorpromazine dose and worsening on the choreoathetosis scale in the lithium group.

The Rapp-Edwards Scale, consisting of items that suggest affective components in schizophrenics, was not statistically associated with study outcome either on clinical variables or in dyskinesia. These negative results may reflect the failure of affective components to exert a major influence on response to lithium in schizophrenics. Alternatively, the Rapp-Edwards items may not identify predictors of lithium response. These items focus on history and social variables rather than target symptoms of affective illness. It might be possible to examine the presence of affective symptoms as possible predictors of lithium response in a larger study.

CONCLUSION

Lithium carbonate was found to be more effective than placebo in reducing dyskinetic movements in chronic schizophrenic outpatients over an eight-week period with antipsychotic dosage held constant. During a variable extended study period of antipsychotic dosage decrease, the lithium effects dissipated. Change in dyskinesia was weakly related to initial antipsychotic dosage. No lithium-placebo differences were found on clinical measures at either eight weeks or at the end of the study. Lithium enabled some patients to remain clinically stable while their neuroleptic dose was reduced by 80 percent, but patients on high neuroleptic doses tended to decompensate despite the addition of lithium.

Overall, the lithium effectiveness in TD showed in the eight-week study is a positive finding which suggests a continued role for lithium as a therapeutic agent for TD. However, the findings of the extended portion of the study cast serious doubt on the major "hope" of this research, namely that lithium might become a substitute for neuroleptics in a sizable minority of patients.

References

Alexander PE, van Kammen DP, Bunney WE: Antipsychotic effect of lithium in schizophrenia. Am J Psychiatry 138:283–287, 1979

Aminoff MJ, Marshall J: Treatment of Huntington's chorea with lithium carbonate. Lancet 1:107–109, 1974

Beitman BD: Tardive dyskinesia reinduced by lithium carbonate. Am J Psychiatry 135:1229–1230, 1978

Biederman J, Lerner Y, Belmaker RH: Combination of lithium carbonate and haloperidol in schizo-affective disorder. Arch Gen Psychiatry 36: 327–333, 1979

Brockington IF, Kendell RE, Kellett JM, et al: Trials of lithium, chlorpromazine, and amitriptyline in schizo-affective patients. Br J Psychiatry 133:162–168, 1978

Cade JFJ: Lithium salts in the treatment of psychotic excitement. Med J Aust 36:349–352, 1949

Carmen JS, Bigelow LB, Wyatt, RJ: Lithium combined with neuroleptics in chronic schizophrenic and schizoaffective patients. J Clin Psychiatry 42:124–127, 1981

Cohen WJ, Cohen NH: Lithium carbonate, haloperidol, and irreversible brain damage. JAMA 230:1283–1287, 1974

Crews EL, Carpenter AE: Lithium-induced aggravation of tardive dyskinesia. Am J Psychiatry 134:933, 1977

Dalen P: Lithium therapy in Huntington's chorea and tardive dyskinesia. Lancet 1:107–108, 1973

Delva N, Letemendia FJJ, Prowse A: Lithium withdrawal trial in chronic schizophrenia. Br J Psychiatry 141:401–406, 1982

Donaldson IM, Cunningham J: Persisting neurologic sequelae of lithium carbonate therapy. Arch Neurol 40:747–751, 1983

Endicott J, Spitzer RL, Fleiss J, et al: The global assessment scale. Arch Gen Psychiatry 33:766–771, 1976

Ereshefsky K, Rubin TN, Friedman S: Treatment of tardive dyskinesia and mania with RBC lithium determinations. Am J Psychiatry 136:570–573, 1979

Gallager DW, Pert A, Bunney WE: Haloperidol-induced presynaptic dopamine supersensitivity is blocked by chronic lithium. Nature 273:309–312, 1978

Gerlach J, Thorsen K, Munkvad I: Effect of lithium on neuroleptic-induced tardive dyskinesia compared with placebo in a double-blind crossover trial. Pharmakopsychiatrie/Neuro-Psychopharmakologie 8:51–56, 1975

Glazer WM, Sheard MH: Relapse in patients with shifting RDC diagnoses treated with lithium alone. J Clin Psychiatry 43:134–136, 1982

Goodnick PJ, Meltzer HY: Effect of subchronic lithium treatment on apomorphine-induced change in prolactin and growth hormone secretion. J Clin Psychopharmacol 3:239–243, 1983

Growe GA, Crayton JW, Klass DB, et al: Lithium in chronic schizophrenia. Am J Psychiatry 136:454–455, 1979

Guy W: ECDEU Assessment Manual for Psychopharmacology. Washington, DC, US Department of Health, Education and Welfare, 1976, p. 534–537

Hamra B, Dunner F, Larson C: Remission of tics with lithium therapy. J Clin Psychiatry 44:73–74, 1983

Hirschowitz J, Casper RV, Garver DL, et al: Lithium response in good prognosis schizophrenia. Am J Psychiatry 137:916–920, 1980

Hussain, MG, Gommersell JD: The use of lithium in the treatment of schizo-affective disorders, in Lithium in Medical Practice. Edited by Johnson FN, Johnson S. Baltimore, University Park Press, 1978

Johnson G: Differential response to lithium carbonate in manic-depressive and schizo-affective disorders. Diseases of the Nervous System 31:613–615, 1970

Jus A, Villeneuve A, Gautier J, et al: Deanol, lithium, and placebo in the treatment of tardive dyskinesia. Neuropsychobiology 4:140–149, 1978

Klawans HL, Weiner WJ, Nausieda PA: The effect of lithium on animal models of tardive dyskinesia. Prog Neuropsychopharmacol 1:53–60, 1977

Leonard DP, Kidson MA, Shannon PJ, et al: Double-blind trial of lithium carbonate and haloperidol in Huntington's chorea. Lancet 2:1208–1209, 1974

Mackay A, Sheppard GP, Sata BK, et al: Failure of lithium treatment in established tardive dyskinesia. Psychol Med 10:583–587, 1980

Overall JE, Gorham DR: The brief psychiatric rating scale. Psychol Rep 10:799, 1962

Pert A, Rosenblatt JE, Siritt C, et al: Long-term treatment with lithium prevents the development of dopamine receptor supersensitivity. Science 201:171–173, 1978

Pickar D, Davis RK: Tardive dyskinesia in younger patients. Am J Psychiatry 135:385–386, 1978

Pope HG, Lipinski JF: Diagnosis in schizophrenia and manic-depressive illness. Arch Gen Psychiatry 35:811–828, 1978

Prakash R, Kelwala S, Ban TA: Neurotoxicity in patients with schizophrenia during lithium therapy. Compr Psychiatry 23:271–273, 1982

Prange AJ, Wilson IC, Morris CE, et al: Preliminary experience with tryptophan and lithium in the treatment of tardive dyskinesia. Psychopharmacol Bull 9:36–37, 1973

Prien RF, Caffey EM, Klett CJ: A comparison of lithium carbonate and chlorpromazine in the treatment of excited schizo-affectives. Arch Gen Psychiatry 27:182–189, 1972

Rapp MS, Edwards P: A high prevalence of affective disorder discovered in a "schizophrenia clinic." Canadian Psychiatric Association Journal 22:181–183, 1977

Reda FA, Escobar JL, Scanlen JM: Lithium carbonate in the treatment of tardive dyskinesia. Am J Psychiatry 132:560–562, 1975

Shopsin B, Johnson G, Gershon S: Neurotoxicity with lithium: differential drug responsiveness. Int Pharmakopsychiatry 5:170–182, 1970

Simpson GM: Tardive dyskinesia. Br J Psychiatry 122:618, 1973

Simpson GM, Branchey MH, Lee JH, et al: Lithium in tardive dyskinesia. Pharmakopsychiatrie Neuro-Psychopharmakologie 9:76–80, 1976

Simpson GM, Lee JH, Zoubok B, et al: A rating scale for tardive dyskinesia. Psychopharmacology 64:171–179, 1979

Small J, Kellams J, Milstein V, et al: A placebo-controlled study of lithium combined with neuroleptics in chronic schizophrenic patients. Am J Psychiatry 132:1315–1317, 1975